THE HOSPICE EXPERIMENT

The Hospice Experiment

EDITED BY

VINCENT MOR, Ph.D.

Director, Center for Gerontology and Health Care Research,
Brown University, and Project Director, National Hospice Study

DAVID S. GREER, M.D.

Dean of Medicine, Brown University,
and Principal Investigator, National Hospice Study

&

ROBERT KASTENBAUM, Ph.D.

Director, Adult Development and Aging Program,
Arizona State University,
and Principal Consultant, National Hospice Study

The Johns Hopkins University Press
Baltimore and London

CB

Second printing, 1989

The Johns Hopkins University Press
701 West 40th Street
Baltimore, Maryland 21211
The Johns Hopkins Press Ltd., London

The paper used in this publication
meets the minimum requirements of American National Standard
for Information Sciences—Permanence of Paper
for Printed Library Materials,
ANSI Z39.48-1984. ∞

This work was supported in part by grants from DHHS/HCFA (no. 99-P-97793/1-0), the
Robert Wood Johnson Foundation, and the John A. Hartford Foundation.

Library of Congress Cataloging-in-Publication Data

The Hospice experiment.

(The Johns Hopkins series in contemporary medicine
and public health)
"This work was supported in part by grants from
DHHS/HCFA Grant no. 99-P-97793/1-0, from the Robert
Wood Johnson Foundation, and the John A. Hartford
Foundation"—T.p. verso.
Bibliography: p.
Includes index.
1. Hospices (Terminal care)—United States.
I. Mor, Vincent. II. Greer, David S. III. Kastenbaum,
Robert. IV Robert Wood Johnson Foundation. V. John
A. Hartford Foundation. VI. Series. [DNLM: 1. Hospices
—United States. 2. Terminal Care. WX 28.6 AA1 H77]
R726.8.H665 1988   362.1'75   87-22580
ISBN 0-8018-3542-9 (alk. paper)

Contents

List of Contributors

RICHARD GOLDBERG, M.D., Associate Professor, Department of Psychiatry and Human Behavior, Brown University, and Psychiatrist-in-Chief, Rhode Island Hospital and Women and Infants Hospital, Providence, R.I.

CLAIRE E. GUTKIN, PH.D., Senior Research Associate, Department of Social Gerontological Research, Hebrew Rehabilitation Center for Aged, Roslindale, Mass.

JEFFREY HIRIS, M.A., Programmer/Analyst, Center for Gerontology and Health Care Research, Brown University

DAVID KIDDER, PH.D., Senior Economist, Abt Associates, Inc., Cambridge, Mass.

LINDA LALIBERTE, J.D., M.S., Research Operations Manager, Center for Gerontology and Health Care Research, Brown University

JOHN N. MORRIS, PH.D., Associate Director, Department of Social Gerontological Research, Hebrew Rehabilitation Center for Aged, Roslindale, Mass.

SYLVIA SHERWOOD, PH.D., Director, Department of Social Gerontological Research, Hebrew Rehabilitation Center for Aged, Roslindale, Mass.

SUSAN M. WRIGHT, B.A., Researcher/Analyst, Office of Institutional Planning, Tufts University

Foreword

In 1979 when the letter arrived advising that our home health agency had been selected as one of the twenty-six hospice programs to serve as demonstration sites in the National Hospice Study (NHS), our hospice acquired a degree of credibility far beyond what we had been able to achieve in many months of difficult discussions with physicians, hospitals, and our own home health staff. The letter spelled survival for our embattled program. The demonstration would fund the services our parent home health agency was currently underwriting and allow us to provide other services we "knew" our patients/families needed. We were absolutely confident the NHS would confirm what we had told members of the lay and health professional community for months: hospice provided better pain management for cancer victims than traditional care; it offered better quality of life to patients and families facing death; and it was a cost-effective alternative to conventional care.

What we did not know, and perhaps could not foresee, was the role the NHS and the demonstration would have in defining American hospice care. The government may not have fully considered the type of "health" providers it would examine when it considered using a scientific evaluation process. About all that was immediately similar about the twenty-six demonstration sites was

Editor's Note: Barbara McCann was a director of one of the original hospice demonstration programs included in the National Hospice Study. Since leaving that position, she was responsible for developing and then implementing quality of care and accreditation guidelines for hospice care at the Joint Commission on Accreditation of Health Care Organizations. She currently serves as the director of that organization's Accreditation Program for Hospice Care and Home Care Development.

our belief in a hospice philosophy of care, a commitment that from a sociocultural perspective now was the time to address better care of the dying either within or outside traditional health care, and the availability of particular interdisciplinary team services that were provided by volunteers or paid staff.

The NHS took this conglomeration of philosophy and services and developed an evaluation model that led both formally and informally to a definition of hospice practice and ultimately the reimbursable model of hospice care in this country. The study appropriately involved the directors from the twenty-six sites on an ongoing basis for dialogue and input. The study authors asked us to answer questions about utilization, our patients, care delivery patterns, and staff qualifications. All of these were issues that hospice as a whole had not formally addressed, nor had we as directors of individual programs addressed these issues beyond the immediate level of day-to-day care. What emerged from the study's need for input was an informal process among the directors that actually worked to forge a consensus definition of the hospice model. Every time an issue arose in which there was a difference in practice among providers, we discussed the reasons, informally came to a judgment about the right way care should be handled in a hospice, and inadvertently through this process, forged more common standards of practice and delivery-system organizations.

A particular example is the NHS effort to examine the type, duration, and purpose of nursing visits. Many of us had not previously considered nursing visits as explicitly as this. In the course of informal discussions, we learned that the community-based home-care programs, or independent hospices, primarily used volunteer nurses who made only two patient visits per day. Those of us from home health agencies were hesitant as we pushed our nurses to make three to four visits a day (a substantial reduction from the expectations of normal home health agency nurses). As the average cost of nursing services was revealed during the study, it was clear that the fewer the visits, the higher the cost. Everyone silently knew that cost-effectiveness was our "ticket" to survival. The nursing visit frequency had to be increased. Faced with this reality and having the funding available from the demonstration to hire staff, some volunteer nurses were replaced with paid staff. The paid staff would make more visits and more efficiently address the increased caseload experienced by almost all of the twenty-six sites following award of the demonstration. The same phenomena also occurred in many sites with regard to bereavement services. After months of struggling with home volunteers and staff providing follow-up, bereavement services were now reimbursable under the demonstration. Many of us used the new funding to hire a professional counselor as a bereavement coordinator. We continued to use volunteers for follow-up, but the counselor could use the reimbursable visits to conduct an assessment, establish a care plan, and introduce the volunteer.

In both instances we all felt that hiring professional staff seemed to be efficient management and utilization of available resources. In retrospect, our decisions initiated the process of professionalization of hospice care. Our changing management style also changed the rules and generalization of the evaluation. The NHS results would be based on programs that used more and more professional staff, not the volunteer-intensive hospice model that reflected the majority of programs across the country. By basing the evaluation on a professional model of hospice care, we may have inadvertently initiated the first step in the demise of the volunteer hospice. The demonstration would become the basis for legislation, licensure regulations, and third-party payment throughout the country. We had set a standard of professional practice that volunteer hospices could not meet and were never created to meet.

The NHS also highlighted the issue of difference in the utilization of inpatient care. Our informal discussions revealed two very different philosophies about the use of inpatient care. The hospital-based programs that had a dedicated hospice unit provided inpatient care more frequently than did the home-care programs. We in the home-based hospice programs listened to descriptions of patients who spent little or no time at home or those who sought the comfort of the unit as death approached. The NHS confirms our perception of a difference in what types of patients need inpatient care. One might attribute the difference perhaps to the patient's choice, but I can't help but wonder if there was not more involved. In the early 1980s patients and families did not know what hospice was except what we told them. In retrospect I can't help but ask how much the locus of the hospice program in the inpatient or home-care setting directly or indirectly affected the patient's choice of setting, our management of care, and ultimately the very patients we admitted to the hospice.

Our hospice *was* home care. We didn't receive referrals unless the doctor or discharge planner knew there was someone at home to care for the patient. We didn't have an inpatient unit, and our goal was to provide the help needed to keep patients at home even through death. That's where they wanted to be—or was it? I distinctly remember one instance in which I finished what I thought was a successful family conference. The middle-aged children who were visiting had read Kübler-Ross and wanted Dad to die at home where he belonged. The elderly wife who had remained very quiet finally shouted into my face, "Don't you understand I can't live here and remember him dead in the living room?" How many times did we give families the message that being at home, staying at home, and dying at home was the right thing to do? Did we always objectively assess the prolonged stress on the primary careperson or the appropriateness from several perspectives of care in the inpatient setting versus the home-care setting? Could we have tried harder to make effective relationships with inpatient facilities before the Medicare legislation forced us to do so? How much did our attitude contribute to defining hospice care as home care in this country? These were all questions we did not debate formally or informally as the cost data came in, which clearly showed that inpatient care reduced the amount of health-care cost savings attributable to hospice. It was clear home care had to be emphasized if we were to be cost effective, which we saw as crucial to having a hospice benefit, receiving payment and recognition, and in the end, preserving our own survival.

The results of the NHS that follow provide us with evidence of clear differences among providers. They painfully, yet straightforwardly, reveal the weaknesses of hospices in America. Although the study data were collected in 1982 and 1983, the profile they present still reflects hospice in America today. Hospice emerges as a viable alternative for terminally ill patients who have primary caregivers and wish to be cared for in the home. For these patients hospice care is cost effective if their length of stay is not too long. The quality of their life will be no worse, or necessarily better, than those who choose to use more inpatient hospice care or conventional care, although the stress experienced by the caregiver may be greater in view of possible prolonged twenty-four-hour home-care responsibilities. Pain management may not be as effective as that provided in the hospital-based programs. Unfortunately, many of these units no longer exist as a result of denials and limitations of reimbursement for inpatient hospice care that have accompanied the introduction of prospective payment for hospitalization.

We must all ask ourselves if the findings of the NHS reflect the hospice we envisioned in America before the demonstration and the introduction of the legislation. Can we truly justify the limited access to inpatient care in terms of quality palliative care? Can we justify that hospice is not reimbursable and therefore not readily available for thousands of individuals who are dying but have no home, no primary caregiver, and a disease other than cancer, which more readily lends itself to a predictable deterioration in six months or less? The NHS results do not allow us to step back eight years to reexamine our formal or informal decisions; they do, however, provide an excellent starting point for a new public policy discussion and hospice provider debate as to what hospices are and whom we can serve.

Barbara A. McCann

Acknowledgments

Hundreds of individuals contributed to the National Hospice Study from its initial conception in 1978 to its conclusion in 1985. Multiple government agencies as well as foundations provided extensive support, both financial and technical, to the design, implementation, and evaluation of the project. A National Advisory Panel was convened and actively worked with us throughout the study, providing advice and expertise in all phases of this complex undertaking. A broad array of consultants ranging in fields from economics to thanatology assisted us in various stages in the planning and then the analysis of the study data. The actual study effort was a composite of the over fifty hospice and conventional-care programs that were the programs studied and the multiple research groups that collaborated to undertake the evaluation. We would like to take this opportunity to enumerate some of the individuals in each of these groups who were so important to bringing the study to fruition.

We benefited from the active involvement of a number of project officers from the funding agencies who did so much initially to shape and conceptualize the project and then to facilitate its implementation. From the Health Care Financing Administration, Richard Yaffe and Lawrence (Spike) Duzor were central in facilitating the project implementation and ensuring that our efforts were incorporated into the regulatory framework at the appropriate times. From the Robert Wood Johnson Foundation, Martita Marx was a driving force in the formulation of the evaluation questions, and Linda Aiken was crucial in ensuring that our results were disseminated. From the John A. Hartford Foundation, in New York City, John Craig and Patricia Drury provided ongoing oversight. From the Social Security Administration, Paula Franklin provided a unique policy perspective for the study.

In addition to the authors of the various chapters of this book, many other investigators and project staff members collaborated with us to undertake the project. From Brown University, Alan Morrison, Donald McClure, and Stuart Geman all provided critical statistical and epidemiological input into the design and particularly the statistical analyses of the study data. Paul Calabresi, Arvin Glicksman, Michael Wiemann, and Robert Fox provided important input into the design of the clinical components of the study. Bruce Foulke, Corrinne Osley, and Susan Allen did much of the day-to-day work organizing data about the hospices and nonhospice study sites. Working with Brown University staff, Robert Teolis and Donald Feragne from Blue Cross and Blue Shield of Rhode Island served as accountants determining the cost of hospice services.

From the Hebrew Rehabilitation Center for Aged, John Peterson and Susan Wright served to coordinate the efforts of our data-collection staff located on the East Coast, and Michael Giarla had the all-important task of designing and managing the project data base. From the Ebenezer Center for Aging, Katherine Gray and Kathy Carroll coordinated the data-collection activities of our staff located in participating Midwestern sites. From Cedars-Sinai Medical Center, Ken Hepburn and Freddi Danner undertook a parallel task in our West Coast participating sites.

Abt Associates, Inc., in Cambridge, Massachusetts, contributed the expertise of a number of analysts in health economics and in the design of the cost data collection and analysis segments of the study. Howard Birnbaum served as a coinvestigator of the study, and Craig Coelen provided crucial support and direct assistance at several times of crisis. Nancy Goodrich, Sally Stearns, Joanne Morse, Chris Saia, and Robert Burke all contributed to the effort throughout the course of the project.

Members of our National Advisory Panel were provocative, insightful, and supportive both as a group and individually: David Hamburg, David Blumenthal, Clifton Gaus, Bradford Gray, Bernard Greenberg, Jeffrey Harris, Jimmie Holland, David Mechanic, Steven Sieverts, Walter Spitzer, Arthur Upton, and Jerome Yates.

The expertise of project staff was supplemented by that of numerous consultants. Beatrice Kastenbaum helped design our patient interviews and training protocols for our data-gathering staff and then helped in the editing of this manuscript. Rachel Schwartz assisted in the organizational analyses in the beginning and again at the end of the study. In addition, the following consultants provided review and comments on the study design: Harold A. Cohen, James Lee, William Scanlon, Harry Sobel, and Stanley Wallack.

Over fifty individuals from all walks of life gave up weeks of their lives to participate in 120 hours of training as data collectors and interviewers and then allowed the work of interacting with dying patients and their families to alter their lives for nearly two years. Without them, all of the careful planning and methodology would have been for naught. They were Maryjane Anderson-

Wurth, Peggy Audley, Jeanne Berglund, Bernadette Blong, Patricia Burke, Kathleen Bystrowski, Jacqueline Cabral, Cynthia Callahan, Lucy Feldman, Martha Floberg, Karen Friedman, Patricia Galloway-Banday, Elizabeth Garlichs, Frida Goldstein-Friend, Betty Gordon, Jacqueline Goyette, Theresa Grieco, Sarah Hanson, Richard Hein, Elizabeth Heun, Shirley Kasten, Sylvia Kenig, William Kittridge, Barbara Lowinger, Carol Mahoney, Linda Mangini, Donna McCarthy, Francis McGuire, Betty Meredith, Michelle Merry, Jason Meyer, Gloria Miranda, Sandra Nash, Cynthia Nelson, Rebecca Picatoste, Patricia Rork, Beverly Ryan, Judith Seipp, Linda Shultz, Selma Slate, Lynn Slifer, Kay Stivlund, Linda Sundstrom, Michael Thomas, G. Timms, Diane Trujillo, William Van Siclen, Pattye Williams, Janet Winston, LaVonne Wontorek, Nancy Wood, and Ray Zischang.

Perhaps most important, our greatest gratitude goes to the patients and families who participated in the study. In giving their time and willingly sharing their intimate feelings and experiences with our field staff, these individuals made it possible to contribute to the shaping of future policy, which was so often their wish.

For the hours of formatting, reference checking, and for all of the compulsive care in the preparation of this manuscript, a special thanks goes to April Krauss, whose attention to detail has been so important.

Finally, this work is presented in memoriam of our esteemed friend and colleague, Michael Pozen, whose invaluable contribution to the study significantly shaped its design. Although he bore innumerable other responsibilities, his efforts on behalf of the study extended far beyond the limitations implicit in his appointed role. Mike's tragic death left us with a great sense of loss.

THE HOSPICE EXPERIMENT

1

The Hospice Experiment: An Alternative in Terminal Care

VINCENT MOR, DAVID S. GREER, AND ROBERT KASTENBAUM

The glory, jest, and riddle of the universe!
— POPE

Alexander Pope was seldom disappointed when surveying the human condition for likely targets. Organized around the pain of his own rejection by society, Pope's misanthropic wit was dedicated to revealing the blemishes and pretenses of others. What irony Pope might have found in the very existence of this book. A few years ago, Americans did everything but die—we went to our great reward, passed on, expired, or were "transferred to Allen Street" (in the argot of Massachusetts General Hospital). That humankind is mortal was a secret withheld from those completing their professional training in medicine, nursing, psychology, and related fields. The concept of *terminal care* was all but unknown. A rare psychologist (e.g., Herman Feifel), sociologist (e.g., Thomas Eliot), or philosopher (e.g., Jacques Choron) would broach the subject at the risk of hostility and ostracism within his own discipline. The establishment (in the form of hospitals, universities, and government agencies) took the official position that the problem was not dying and death but rather the tactless impulse some people had in bringing up such unpleasant and unproductive topics.

Well might Pope have pondered our resistance to acknowledging the more horizontal facts of life. For a being "created half to rise and half to fall," *Homo americanus* had a distinct aversion to open discourse regarding either sex or death. How tempting a target would Pope have noted in our vertical strivings, ever onward and upward, while pretending that horizontality is not also a human posture, and one that rounds every mortal life. The "chaos of thought and passion, all confused; Still by himself abused" that Pope addressed in his *Essay on Man* would have abundant new examples awaiting dissection.

Perhaps the eighteenth-century poet would find his prime jest in the fact that the same establishment for which death had been so long a taboo subject (Feifel

1963) has now enacted legislation, issued directives, and insisted on scientific evaluation of alternative modalities for terminal care. The federal government in particular has assumed the role of benefactor and regulator for an activity once steadfastly ignored. Pope might also see in this transformation something of the glory of our flawed species, "a being darkly wise, and rudely great."

It is the riddle of the hospice movement, however, that most concerns us here. The riddle has several interrelated components. How and why did American society develop its studied neglect of dying and death? What forces converged to challenge this attitude? How did the hospice alternative develop so rapidly once it gained a foothold? These past-oriented questions lead directly to issues bearing upon the future of the hospice movement. Has the hospice approach actually provided a clear-cut alternative to traditional care of the terminally ill person? If so, is this alternative making an appreciable difference in the quality of life for patients and families? And will hospices prove viable in the American health-care system, with its entrenched attitudes and cost-driven pressures?

Conceivably, hospice care could succeed "for all the wrong reasons." It might, for example, prove effective as a cost-reduction mechanism in terminal care but offer little of the hoped-for benefit in quality of life for patients and families. An even more extreme outcome could be envisioned: in practice, perhaps hospice care actually results in *less* adequate care but does save money. It is also conceivable that quite the opposite situation might prevail. The hospice alternative might fail to survive, even if the quality of care proved demonstrably superior, if it also proved too costly in the opinion of decision makers. The *timing* of the hospice movement might also prove critical: perhaps this development was facilitated by a transient set of circumstances whose temporary support will soon be replaced by indifference or even hostility toward such an innovative program. Consideration, then, cannot be limited to any one realm but must be given to such varied topics as dominant sociocultural attitudes; response to changing environmental, economic, and political circumstances; expectations regarding terminal care; the actual operation and achievements of hospice organizations; and their place both in the health-care system and society in general.

This book presents the results of the most extensive study yet undertaken of hospice care in the United States. The specific purposes, methods, and findings are presented in a fairly detailed manner. In this chapter, however, we attempt to describe and interpret the scene upon which hospice care (and this study) made its appearance. The tools of multivariate statistical analysis, so strenuously put to work in the study itself, are not well suited for the present task. Instead, we must rely upon observations made by ourselves and others who played various roles in this scene as it unfolded over recent years. The following observations, then, have no claim on being complete or definitive but simply offer a perspective on the emergence of hospices in the United States.

How Americans View Death

The hospice movement is both an approach to terminal care and a social movement. Attention will be given first to death-related attitudes and practices in the United States prior to the establishment of hospice programs, followed by an exploration of hospice care as a spontaneous social movement.

Of greatest interest here are changes in the American way of death (Mitford 1963) since the end of World War II. It should be understood, however, that recent developments are by no means independent of earlier historical trends (Farrell 1982; Stannard 1977). Death-related attitudes and practices existed in colonial times and have continued to change throughout the Federalist period, the War between the States, the settlement of the West, and the peak years of immigration. The definitive story of our heritage has yet to be told. It would have to take into account such events and factors as the near-extermination experiences of Puritan settlers, the genocidal onslaught against Native Americans, the sulphur-and-brimstone period of pulpit oratory, the unprecedented violence and lingering sorrows of the conflict between the Blue and the Gray, the high mortality rate among children and young mothers, and much else.

If one theme from America's past were to be selected for its connection with contemporary death attitudes, it might well be the emphasis on a better life through hard work and "progress." Grace, salvation, and the kingdom of heaven remained important symbolic values, but the new land also held promise for success here and now. In the minds of many there was an implicit connection between material progress and moral worth. The good person worked hard and enjoyed rewards here *and* hereafter. Fear and grief accompanied the intrusions of death into personal lives (Rosenblatt 1983), but this was not usually communicated through the public stance of confidence in the future. The nation was expanding, growing ever more powerful, with abundant opportunities for the resourceful and hardworking. The wheels of industry were turning, the West was being won, and God obviously had a special interest in America's material and spiritual destiny. "Feeling your oats!" became a popular expression of national zest and optimism. Death seemed quite out of place in this bustling, idealistic, future-striving, adolescent America. Some residuals of this heady time will be noted below as we survey more recent phases in America's view of death.

Institutional Denial

Superficially, there was a massive return to "normality" at the end of World War II. The fact of decisive victory added to the sense of relief that a period of danger, deprivation, and separation had passed. Perhaps death, too, could be left on the battlefields, and life could reconstitute its continuity and promise.

Examinations of American attitudes toward death in the immediate post–World War II years suggested that a pattern of *institutional denial* existed. As distinguished from the psychodynamic mechanism of denial, the institutional form is characteristic of social groups and enfranchised organizations rather than individuals attempting to cope privately with unbearable anxiety (Kastenbaum 1986). The distraught man talking to the corpse of his dead wife as though she were still alive has for the moment allowed his sense of reality to falter under the pressure of extreme stress. In a short time he will probably have discovered other ways to respond and will no longer need to invoke this primitive defense reaction. Institutional denial is a rather different matter. The physician who told a dying man "You're doing fine. You'll be out of here in no time" was not necessarily exhibiting individual psychopathological behavior. He was simply playing his role in maintaining the applicable norms. The famous teaching hospital whose staff "transferred" patients to "Allen Street" instead of acknowledging their deaths was not desperately attempting to control a surge of personal anxiety but, again, was merely doing its part to prevent open acknowledgment of death. Sustained by the cooperative efforts of so many functionaries in the system, institutional denial can be more powerful and enduring than the frantic efforts of a beleaguered individual.

Seemingly unaffected by the recent war experience, Americans continued to avoid acknowledgment of dying and death under most circumstances (violent death remained, as ever, a subject of fascination). People whose work brought them into occasional contact with death—physicians, nurses, ministers, funeral directors, attorneys, and life insurance salesmen—all had perfected little "routines" that enabled them to do their jobs without coming too close and demonstrating their vulnerability. ("The guy spoke to us more than two hours, trying to sell us more life insurance. First it was comical, then I just got sore at him because he just couldn't bring himself to say why it is anyone needs 'life' insurance." "Then the chaplain came in, and he did his little song and dance, and he scooted out before my sister even had a chance to say anything to him. And we thought *we* were the nervous ones!") The educational system held its silence from kindergarten through professional schools, and the powerful new television medium joined its radio and print brethren in ignoring "natural" (nonviolent) dying and death. It was only in the next phase of social response to death, however, that the characteristics and extent of institutional denial came to light.

Recognizing the Taboo

The business-as-usual orientation following World War II was not as complete and unanimous as it might have appeared on the surface. Perhaps a great many people now had doubts occasioned by their experiences with death, destruction, and social upheaval. If these doubts were most often kept to one's self, there were some keen observers and articulate writers who ventured to express themselves. Existential philosophy and psychology drifted over from war-devastated Europe (Kaufmann 1959) and found some intellectual resonance here. Far from a monolithic or even a consistent school of philosophy, existentialism did introduce questions about life and death that had seldom arisen to perturb the pragmatic, accomplishing, denying Americans.

The American version of postwar revisionary thinking did not usually linger in the philosophical domain. What developed instead was a new critical tradition focusing on specific problems and inequities. Beginning in the 1950s and becoming increasingly powerful through the 1960s, these critiques provided a catalog of the incongruous, the ineffective, the ignorant, and the outrageous. Viewed now in retrospect, the critics seem to have maintained a certain distance from their subject matter, as though standing in the doorway and urgently asking others to come and see what they had seen. The phase of the active reformer was not yet at hand: we had first to open our eyes to the fact that our eyes had been for so long closed.

Clinical psychologist Herman Feifel broke through several barriers that had stood in the way of death awareness among professionals and scientists. His studies of death attitudes were perhaps more important for the simple fact that they had been completed and published than for the particular results obtained. He managed to persuade a major scientific organization, the American Psychological Association, to schedule a symposium on death and dying. This symposium attracted such a large and involved audience that the day of a psychology-without-death had finally come to an end. Of broader impact was his *Meaning of Death* (1959), a book that had to overcome the hesitations and anxieties of a major publisher who until almost the last minute tried to delete the word *death* from the title. *Time* magazine, recognizing that this book represented a breakthrough, devoted its medicine section to a favorable review. For the first time in decades, Americans could pick up a popular periodical and read a levelheaded discussion of dying and death on the contemporary scene. Featuring a contribution by the eminent psychoanalyst Carl C. Jung, as well as others by a variety of clinicians and social scientists, *The Meaning of Death* presented material suggesting not only that Americans strenuously resisted awareness of death but also that this attitude had an adverse effect on interpersonal relationships and professional caregiving. Aronson's "Treatment of the Dying Person" (1959) and Kasper's "The Doctor and Death" (1959) pointed out areas of concern that would later become the nucleus of grass-roots advocacy for an alternative in terminal care. Gardner Murphy, one of the nation's most respected psychologists, suggested in Feifel's *The Meaning of Death* (1959) that death was becoming increasingly more difficult to integrate into the lives of both the individual and society at large because impersonal killing had shown itself to be a hallmark of the twentieth century while at the same time belief in afterlife was continuing to decline. If death no longer made much sense or opened the door to the kingdom of heaven, then it was more attractive than ever to avoid death-related thoughts and feelings whenever possible.

From this point forward there would be the gradual creation of a body of scholarly and professional studies centering on dying and death. The topic remained unusual but steadily gained acceptance. Of far greater public influence, however, were books offered by popular writers with the ability to entertain as well as inform. Two British writers amused and aroused American sensibilities with books portraying the funeral industry. Evelyn Waugh's *Loved One* (1948) was a witty and slightly bizarre parody of behind-the-scenes life among funeral directors that reached American readers a decade after its appearance in Britain. Jessica Mitford's *American Way of Death* (1963) was a nonfiction best-seller, expressing outrage at the alleged manipulation of American consumers by those who merchandise funerals. Both books had not only the virtue of attractive writing but also that of encouraging people to deal with some aspects of death by offering an immediate emotional reward (amusement and righteous indignation). Furthermore, neither book required the reader to enter the most threatening emotional territory—fear of personal dying and death. One could stand at a safe distance, chuckling over Miss Thanatopsis's efforts to construct philosophical smile number seven on the visage of the deceased or agreeing with Mitford that funeral directors sometimes pursued the profit motive too vigorously. (Superior and better-balanced books on the funeral industry, such as Bowman's *American Funeral* [1959], enjoyed but a fraction of the readership.) The Waugh and Mitford books encouraged further writings and discussions in which some of death's reality and anxiety could be acknowledged as long as reassuringly embedded in a literary context. The fact that books dealing with death could be very profitable also began to impress itself on some media executives, preparing the way for subsequent ventures.

By the end of the 1960s one could find a lively countertrend in which American death-related attitudes and practices were subjected to critical examination, and long-standing assumptions were replaced by empirical research (e.g., the axiom that dying people don't want to talk about death quickly dissolved as they were given the opportunity to do so). Nevertheless, very little had been accomplished in the actual care of dying people and their families. A challenge had been sounded, but the denial, the impersonality, and the suffering continued in all but the most exceptional settings.

Recognizing the Pain

Recognizing the taboo was perhaps a necessary preliminary phase in preparing the way for the hospice alternative. Obviously, however, something was still lacking in public awareness and response. That "something" transfigured the scene with the publication of Elizabeth Kübler-Ross's *On Death and Dying* (1969). It was again a fortuitous combination of media exposure and timely substance that made the difference. A decade after *Time* had featured Feifel's book, *Life* discovered that a psychiatrist in a suburban Chicago hospital had dared to interview dying patients and discuss them in teaching sessions with other staff members. This pictorial story, again a sympathetic treatment, introduced America to the dying person. Studies of death attitudes and critiques of funeral practices had neither the immediacy nor the power of seeing a person, much like ourselves, but confronting a terminal illness.

The death-awareness movement now had an identifiable and charismatic individual at its core. Kübler-Ross proved to be a highly effective speaker and soon was making personal appearances throughout the nation. Unburdened by the methodological cautions of academia and relatively free of psychiatric jargon, she communicated simply and directly. Kübler-Ross spoke of particular people facing death and at times conducted interviews in front of the audience. Furthermore, by her own example she made it clear that the dying person did not have to remain in social isolation. She could and did sit down with dying people—providing for many in her audience the first such example.

Those who attended Kübler-Ross lectures and workshops in the early 1970s will have no difficulty remembering the emotional atmosphere. Many people felt deeply touched by her presentations. Particularly significant was the frequent reaction on the part of nurses. After years of stressful experience with dying patients, nurses at last had found somebody who recognized their pain, the sorrows they had been given no opportunity to express. It was not unusual for nurses (as well as some others) to weep openly. They were no longer alone with the anguish so often experienced while trying to "act professional" with dying patients. In turn, those who had heard and read Kübler-Ross would often try to emulate her, drawing others into the widening and deepening dialogue. The substance of the discussion—including the soon-famous "five stages of dying"—was for the moment less important than the fact that pain had been recognized and given some relief through open expression.

Death Talk

Once America had been given permission to talk about death, it seemed to some observers that we would never stop. Eventually some wry observers suggested that we were trying to talk death to death. The first wave of "death talk" followed as a natural consequence of exposure to the writings and lectures of Kübler-Ross and other pioneers. Under other circumstances this new dialogue might have led to a gradually improved integration of death-related topics into the American consciousness. It would no longer be a taboo topic but instead would take its place among the many other concerns that people share with those closest to them. This, however, is not what happened. Although a slower, more natural process of increasing death awareness did occur in some settings, the trajectory was much swifter on the national level.

The media "discovered" death with a vengeance. The Sunday supplement, the family-oriented magazine, the television special, and, of course, the talk shows, vied with each other to present death-oriented material. These presentations varied greatly in substance and quality. We can recall a number of thoughtful and accurate presentations in print and on the air. The element of sensationalism was also in evidence, however—we can remember more than one talk show host who was more interested in the shock value of the subject than in thoughtful discussion.

For a short but eventful period of time, death became the media's darling. This exaggerated attention gave rise to a perhaps inevitable backlash. People began to complain of having heart-rending death for radio breakfast, television supper, and after-dinner movie. There was another consequence, less known to the general public. People with a particular interest in death—caregivers, researchers, and those with commercial motivations—tended to assume that America had made a decisive move toward acceptance. There would now be widespread support for innovative programs, for systematic studies, or for profitable death-related services and ventures. These expectations soon were dashed as death talk swiftly reached its peak and then declined. The media had had its fling with death and was moving on to other "discoveries."

Death education did gain and retain a foothold, especially at the college level, but the more ambitious attempts along this line seldom had a lasting success. There was more receptivity than before, but the old resistance was still there under the surface. Research into various aspects of dying and death continued, but no large-scale or breakthrough studies appeared (nor did more ample financial support become available for such research). Individuals who thought that the new death awareness would lead to a market for such services as cryonic suspension ("Freeze—wait—reanimate!") were sorely disappointed by the meager response.

There were valuable and lasting gains from the death-talk phase but also much ephemera and many false starts. Media overkill was not the most fundamental reason for the limited yield of death talk. Simply put, talk was not enough. An effective, viable action program was needed. Without a vehicle for concerted effort, the overall death-awareness movement might have gradually lost its impetus, leaving a heightened sensitivity but little else in its wake.

The Grassroots Context of Hospice Development

The hospice approach to terminal care has emerged as the major instrumentality of the death-awareness movement. Hospice care picked up where sensitivity and talk left off. The general history of the international hospice movement has been well told elsewhere (Stoddard 1978). Here our focus is upon hospice care as the outcome of a grass-roots social movement in the United States and some of the associated conditions and consequences. It will be seen that this movement is still very much in motion and has perhaps yet to acquire its definitive form and scope.

The Hospice Vision

America entered the 1970s without a single hospice program. A recent estimate is that approximately 1,500 programs are functioning in the United States, with nearly another 200 in Canada (Lamers 1986). This rapid growth was accomplished largely by private citizens who saw in the hospice movement a significantly different approach to terminal care. Hospice care was not imposed upon communities and caregivers by pressure or regulation from higher government echelons. It was—and to some extent remains—an idea, a vision that recruited the enthusiasm of both lay people and professionals.

What is this idea whose time ripened so propitiously? The bare outlines of the hospice approach were encapsulated in recommendations made by an international task force in 1975 whose membership included Dame Cicely Saunders, founder-director of the pioneering St. Christopher's Hospice (London). The task force proposed two very basic guidelines for care: (1) the terminally ill person's own preferences and life-style must be taken into account in all decision making; and (2) family members and other caregivers also have legitimate needs and interests that must be taken into consideration (Kastenbaum 1975). Starting from this broad perspective, then, one would not expect patients and their families to accept the treatment styles and preferences of the medical establishment. On the contrary, it is "the system" that must find ways to respect the distinctive circumstances and needs of every individual facing death. Furthermore, the patient is not to be "processed" as though an isolated entity. The individual's social integrity must also be respected and everything possible done to support the existing fabric of interpersonal relationships. Simple though these principles may appear, they signaled a revolutionary approach in terminal care. Fulfillment of the hospice vision would preclude depersonalizing a person as a "colon," "head-neck," or "lung" to be managed according to local protocol. Each patient would be appreciated instead as a total person who had vital connections to other people and who should not be expected to surrender values and preferences developed over a lifetime in order to die in a manner convenient to the system.

More specifically, the task force declared that remission of symptoms is a major treatment goal. It was not acceptable to abandon comfort-giving procedures when nothing more could be done to reverse the terminal course. That the reduction of physical and mental distress had to be emphasized as a key goal of treatment reminds us that this course of action could not be taken for granted in the prehospice milieu. Pain control received special attention. A frequent criticism of traditional management of terminal care had been the failure to provide consistent relief from pain. The hospice vision centered on a person who was not distracted by suffering and the fear of suffering and therefore could still think clearly and maintain significant interpersonal relationships. Another basic goal was for the patient to have a sense of basic trust and security in his or her environment. In a word, the person should feel *safe*. This is possible only when there is a consistent and dependable plan of care maintained by people who really do care. Particular attention was given to the importance of the final days and hours. The task force urged that opportunities should be provided for leave-taking with the people most important to the patient. This guideline would require the abandonment of restricted visiting privileges in the traditional hospital and the availability of privacy within an environment conducive to intimate sharings. Similarly, it was recommended that opportunities be provided for experiencing the final moments in a way that is meaningful to the particular individual.

The hospice vision, then, represented a departure from the types of situations that had been increasingly criticized—the patient either subjected to invasive but useless medical procedures or virtually abandoned. With the hospice approach there should never be either abandonment or a driven effort to try every device and maneuver known to medicine. Another radical departure was the role of family and friends. Traditional management of terminal illness had little place for family members. As one woman recalled, "It was as though I was not there at all, and as though Charlie belonged to them. I was only his wife and nobody cared about that. They were so busy being busy!" By contrast, hospice care was intended to draw upon the love and support of people closest to the dying person. It was to provide technical and social support to help preserve existing relationships, not to be the faceless establishment that takes over other people's lives. Several additional guidelines recognized that family members had legitimate rights and needs in the terminal-care situation and that the same held true of all staff and volunteers as well. One of these guidelines is particularly interesting in its contrast with traditional practices at the time: *A mutual support network should exist among the staff, encompassing both the technical and socioemotional dimensions of working with the terminally ill* (Kastenbaum 1975).

Evidence that this philosophy could work in practice was provided most effectively by St. Christopher's Hospice. Visitors from the United States and other nations were able to see the ideas in action for themselves. One could be impressed by the design of the hospice facility itself, the skill of the medical and nursing staffs in alleviating pain and other symptoms, the reassuring presence of family and volunteers, and the overall atmosphere of serenity. The anxiety of uncontrolled pain and the haunted look of isolation and rejection was seldom if ever observed. A much more common scene would be spouse and patient taking tea together and chatting with a nurse or volunteer. Only the hastiest and least attentive visitor, however, would come away with the impression that the hospice was the physical facility and its staff. Dr. Saunders would make it clear that the hospice was a philosophy and program of care, not a physical facility. The home-care program was also at the core of hospice functioning. People remained in their own homes as long as desired and feasible. Some received the benefits of hospice expertise and support without ever entering the facility; others moved several times between home and facility. The point was to provide a continuity of care regardless of location.

There was at least some existing reality, then, to support the hospice vision. It was by no means certain, however, that the hospice concept could be imported successfully to the United States, where the economics of health care and many other factors were dissimilar. Perhaps hospice care would prove to be a good idea that could flourish only under rather special circumstances, including the leadership of such an exceptionally able and persuasive person as Dr. Saunders.

The Growth of Hospice Care in the United States

Obviously, the hospice movement did take root in the United States and Canada despite numerous difficulties. Sympathetic media attention followed the development and establishment of America's first hospice, in New Haven, Connecticut. After strenuous efforts by a consortium of professionals and lay people, the project won the support of both local and federal authorities. When it opened in 1974, with a home-care program and a forty-four-bed inpatient facility, America had its own centerpiece for the hospice vision. (The early history of the New Haven Hospice is recounted by Lack and Buckingham 1978.)

This first step, however, did not guarantee that other groups of interested citizens would be equally successful in other communities. Enthusiasm for the new endeavor recruited many people who had already been active in the death-awareness movement but also others who were attracted by the opportunity to add something valuable to their own communities. Local circumstances varied greatly in the receptivity accorded to hospice projects. The medical community, for example, might become a powerful advocate of hospices in one region but prove a reluctant, even resistant force in another—the difference sometimes coming down to the attitudes of one or two key individuals.

Hospice advocates not only had to develop positive collaborations with the entire spectrum of human-services providers in their particular areas but also uncover sources of funding. There was no well-established system for funding care for the terminally ill—the concept itself still needed to be conveyed persuasively to an establishment oriented strongly toward spending money only in the quest of cures.

Furthermore, the growth of hospice care in North America was handicapped at first by lack of agreement as to the most desirable scope, organization, and operational status. This was an important question to resolve—not only for the internal functioning of hospice organizations, but also for presentation of the hospice vision to prospective clients, staff, volunteers, and funding agencies. The New Haven Hospice recognized this need and sponsored a meeting for American and Canadian hospice advocates. From this meeting eventually emerged the National Hospice Organization (NHO). Taking the international task force guidelines as a starting point, the embryonic NHO developed a more detailed set of proposed standards and criteria (NHO 1981). This document preserved and extended a continuity of philosophy that had been inherent in St. Christopher's Hospice as well as the task force recommendations.

These standards and criteria received enough dissemination and favorable reaction that they became part of existing regulations in the Medicare benefit provision (Section 122, Tax Equity and Fiscal Responsibility Act [TEFRA] of 1982) that offers reimbursement for participating hospice programs in the United States. One finds essentially the same core points whether reading the TEFRA document or NHO's standards:

- Health care and services are provided to terminally ill patients and their families.
- The patient, the patient's family, and other persons essential to the patient's life comprise the unit of care. The "hospice patient's family" refers to the patient's immediate relatives; individuals with significant personal ties may be designated as the patient's "family" by mutual agreement among the patient, the individual, and the hospice organization.
- Inpatient and home-care services are closely integrated to ensure continuity and coordination of care.
- Care is available seven days a week, twenty-four hours a day.
- Care is planned and provided by a medically supervised interdisciplinary team composed of several individuals with appropriate skills. The team members work together to plan and provide services that will secure the physical, emotional, and spiritual welfare of the patient and his or her family.
- Palliative and supportive care is directed at allaying the physical and emotional discomfort associated with terminal illness.
- Bereavement services are available and may include follow-up visits and support of the family after the patient dies.
- An educational program is available with two components: (1) educating the patient, family, and interdisciplinary team concerning death and dying, and (2) teaching the family to care for the patient at home.
- Volunteers play an important role in the provision of care.

This configuration has become the working model of the full-service hospice in the United States. Not all participants in the hospice movement agree with this approach, however. One can still find organizations that offer only a partial array of the above services. First NHO and then the federal government selected the hospice model that provided the most extensive range of services and required the most extensive accountability for these services. It should be kept in mind, though, that differences in opinion still exist and, moreover, that some organizations are offering limited service until they can obtain sufficient resources to develop the complete spectrum described above.

Some Forces Conducive to the Growth of the Hospice Movement

How did the hospice movement come this far in so short a time? A good part of the answer must be found in the articulate and persistent advocacy by citizens, both lay and professional, who saw in this program the opportunity to bring comfort where too often anxiety and despair had reigned. It is probable, however, that other synergistic processes were also at work. Although it may be decades before the hospice movement can be put into a balanced perspective, certain contributing processes can be identified at this time (Kastenbaum, in press):

Consumerism. The growth of the consumer movement in the United States, catalyzed by Ralph Nader's attack on the automobile industry, provided a context of readiness for hospice advocacy. The consumer movement quickly spread from its initial focus and altered the relationship between seller and purchaser throughout society. Human services did not long remain exempt. Physicians, attorneys, and other professionals (themselves often participants in the consumers' rights movement) found themselves dealing with a more critical and demanding clientele. Even such "traditionally traditional" fields as the banking industry began to adjust themselves to clients who were not necessarily willing to accept whatever it was the establishment had to offer. The grass-roots movement that selected hospice care as one of its most innovative advocacies also made some impression on the rights of health- and human-services consumers in general. Had the hospice movement been imported a few years earlier it might not have fared nearly so well in a milieu that still supported relatively rigid and predictable interactions between provider and consumer.

Naturalism. Marshall McLuhan's singularly awkward term *retribalization* could also be applied to this facet of the changing scene. Family values were given renewed emphasis, and everybody was suddenly "involved" in "relationships." Organic foods, the "natural look," and wider citizen participation in environmental conservation efforts typified an attitude that was new in its broad appeal if not unprecedented in its substance. The new naturalism was seen by some observers as a reaction against the consequences of excessive individualism, competition, and rampant technological change. Again, the hospice movement was congruent. In its rejection of unnecessary medical technology and its effort to replace impersonal management with intimate, loving care, the hospice movement provided an excellent example for the new naturalism. Providing sensitive terminal care could be seen as one of the most basic ways for family and friends to express togetherness in what was perceived as an otherwise hectic and unfeeling society.

Furthermore, "progress" had become for some a hollow or even negative phrase because of its association with pollution, unemployment, and other fallouts of the industrial enterprise. The bright future envisioned by the immigrant and the feisty opportunist in past generations was no longer in prospect. Death, then, could not be so easily accommodated within an optimistic master plan. If some other kind of accommodation had to be made with dying and death, then perhaps hospice care was the best prospect around.

Holism.   Specialization had brought many advantages to industry, the sciences, the professions, and the population in general. By the time the hospice movement made its appearance in the United States, however, there was already a larger reaction against the fragmenting of human life. Many physicians and other health- and human-services providers found holistic approaches more personally satisfying and, at times, more instrumentally effective as well. "Treating the whole person" had already become a cliché, but now more people were convinced that this was actually the superior approach to cultivate. The interdisciplinary character of hospice care and its encompassing of patient, family, volunteer, and professional caregiver into a unified psychosocial field were very much in keeping with holistic philosophy. The hospice movement might have had a much more difficult obstacle course to negotiate were there not a number of professionals who had already convinced themselves that holism was preferable to the fragmentation of people and services.

Discovering the Total Life Span.   Dying and death had not been the only significant phenomena neglected by society. Little attention had been given to aging and the aged. In fact, most courses on human development closed their books at the end of adolescence. During the same years in which the hospice movement entered the scene there was also a vigorous awakening to the total life span. The new subdiscipline of life-span human development emerged and quickly became important both in academia and in community applications. It is not likely a coincidence that textbook writers were frantically converting to a life-span approach with abundant attention to aging at the same time that hospice legislation was moving forward. On many levels the American public was beginning to take a more encompassing view of life—life with aging and death no longer excluded.

Cost Containment. A very different perspective was also becoming increasingly important. Did America have the ability—and the willingness—to pay its mounting health and social program costs? Concerns about the escalating national debt, unfavorable balance of trade, reduced growth (gross national product), and other financial indicators led policy makers to look for ways to reduce obligations. The health-care system became one of the prime sources of concern. Treatment was becoming ever more expensive, and every year a new echelon crossed the symbolic threshold to age sixty-five and a decade or more of expensive health maintenance. More and more talk was heard of "cost containment" and "the bottom line." When the hospice movement knocked on the door, then, there was already a sense of urgency to discover some means of slowing the growth of health-related services. Since everybody dies, perhaps hospices could hold the costs down and thereby not only save some money but also serve as a model to the rest of the health- and human-services industry. An economist might not know or care much about hospice philosophy, but if the projections suggested that money could be saved . . .

These are but a few of the forces that were at work as the hospice movement established itself in the United States. These and other forces will continue to affect the hospice movement. Some further aspects will be considered in chapters 12 and 13.

A National Hospice Demonstration Project

The National Hospice Study (NHS) is an attempt by representatives of the scientific community to objectively evaluate the success of the hospice mission in the United States. The NHS was designed to assess whether hospice care functions according to its own philosophy and attains its stated goals, whether it is indeed superior to conventional care, and, if so, how. The NHS was mandated by the Health Care Financing Administration to answer these questions as adequately as possible and to provide Congress and the Executive Branch with a data base for hospice policy formulation. The study proved to be complex in planning, execution, and analysis. It is the task of this book to communicate what was learned and to point out what remains to be learned.

Even Pope, that prize misanthrope, might have at last decided that this effort was right and proper, having enjoined us to:

Know then thyself, presume not God to scan,
The proper study of mankind is man.

And might he not also have discovered in this venture a suitable illustration for perhaps the most optimistic line ever to be penned by a confirmed pessimist?

Hope springs eternal in the human breast.

2

Participating Hospices and the Patients They Serve

VINCENT MOR

The hospice movement has come to be a significant force in the United States since the mid-1970s. Estimates from the National Hospice Organization (NHO) suggest that there are over a thousand hospices across the country that in 1984 were estimated to have served some hundred thousand patients (NHO *Newsletter*, January 1985). Three basic models of hospice organization structures have evolved, each with numerous variations. These three models are: (1) hospices affiliated with hospitals, with or without a home-care component, (2) hospices affiliated with preexisting home health agencies without their own inpatient unit, and (3) hospices that emerged as organizations exclusively serving terminal patients, with or without a special inpatient unit. More recent variations include nursing homes, replacing the hospital as the parent provider, and quasi-independent coordinating groups that create hospice programs from the collaborative efforts of existing agencies.

The National Hospice Study Demonstration project, at the time it was initiated by the Health Care Financing Administration (HCFA), sought to select hospices from each of the three types of agencies described above. Indeed, in selecting hospices that applied for the demonstration program, HCFA used hospice type as a major factor in selecting the 26 demonstration projects from the 233 applicants. They wanted to ensure that the study would be able to document differences in these types of organizations, how they respond to the availability of special reimbursement, and how they provide care to the patients and families they serve. Insofar as hospices were still an evolving form of health-care agency, HCFA was interested in observing the natural variation in organizational structure that had evolved from the hospice movement. In order to be consistent with the emphasis HCFA placed upon organizational type in selecting demonstration hospices, the evaluation team also used this criterion in selecting nondemonstration hospices. A total of fourteen nondemonstration hospices were selected for the study in proportions that approximated those of demonstration hospices vis-à-vis hospice type.

The current chapter describes the National Hospice Study (NHS) hospices and the patients they serve. This description should provide a useful backdrop to understanding the research methodology used to test the effect of hospice care on patients' quality of life and health-care costs, as well as the results of the many analyses conducted and how we interpreted them for policy purposes. A more detailed discussion of the process by which the sites were selected and the criteria used to do so is presented in the next chapter. For the present chapter, the qualitative and quantitative descriptions of the hospices are based upon all data assembled about the hospices throughout the course of the NHS and not just descriptions of their state prior to the study.

A Portrait of Three American Hospices

The National Hospice Organization's 1985 directory of hospices lists 27 percent of over 1,000 hospices as being affiliated with hospitals, 19 percent affiliated with existing home health agencies, 41 percent independent (providing exclusively hospice care), and 12 percent that are coalitions of multiple agencies. The NHS sample of 40 hospices, 26 demonstration and 14 nondemonstration, represented the three major types of hospices that exist in the United States. Before describing these hospices in terms of their sizes, staffing patterns, and the patients whom they serve, it may be helpful to have a more qualitative synopsis of each type of hospice that can guide the reader through the more quantitative descriptions. The following descriptions of "typical" hospices of each type are composites of those studied in the NHS.

A *hospital hospice* has eight dedicated beds in a converted wing of a 500-bed general hospital. The staff consist of an administrator, social worker, minister, nursing director, staff nurses (few aides are used), and a medical director. There is a limited home-care program consisting of a single coordinator on the staff of the hospital's home-care department. There are few volunteers, and although separate from the hospital's regular volunteer program, they are engaged in similar activities. The hospital's medical staff is divided on the value of hospice care; some are strongly committed to it, while others never refer their patients. Hospital hospice patients have a median survival in the hospice of only thirty days; 25 percent survive less than ten days. Most of the short-stay patients spend their entire hospice stay in the inpatient unit. In general, the preference is to admit terminal patients to the hospice ward rather than treat them at home.

A *hospice home health program* is a special unit of an urban/suburban Visiting Nurse Association. It is staffed almost entirely by nurses, with the addition of a single social worker and an administrative coordinator; a part-time medical director is employed under contract. Aides and homemakers, who provide the bulk of care to patients at home, are assigned from the pool employed by the agency. There is a small volunteer program with a volunteer coordinator. Referrals come largely from the agency's existing network of discharge planners placed in area hospitals. Most patients are internally transferred from the regular home health service or are admitted to hospice care at the time of their discharge from a hospital. Almost all have intact homes with family helpers.

Independent hospice programs began as a small group of volunteers, lay and professional, committed to changing the pattern of care for the terminally ill. Initially, funding from local foundations, bequests, and other gifts made it possible to hire a coordinator and to formalize a relationship to the local visiting nurse association and hospital. In time, with the potential for Medicare certification and reimbursement, staffs were hired, and both the number of patients served and the amount of service provided increased. Nurses, social workers, supervisory staff, volunteers, a minister, and a clerical staff now comprise the organization. Plans are under way to build an inpatient unit, but currently inpatient services are provided under arrangement with a local hospital. The volunteer program has over a hundred active volunteers involved in direct patient care and administrative functions under the direction of a full-time volunteer coordinator. Patients are frequently referred by family, friends, or initiate contact on their own. Family support is generally very strong.

During the course of the project, it became clear to us that the differential availability of inpatient beds provided another useful way of classifying hospices. We observed that freestanding hospices began to resemble more traditional home health agencies as they became larger and encountered issues of staffing, productivity, and clinical control of care. Additionally, home-care hospices behaved like those affiliated with home health agencies in their tendency not to utilize inpatient settings. By contrast, those few freestanding hospices that had their own inpatient units tended to use inpatient settings about as much as their hospital-affiliated counterparts. Because differences in outcome experienced by hospice patients may be closely related to differential patterns of care, we classified hospice organizations as home care (HC) versus hospital based (HB) on the basis of availability or nonavailability of beds. The HC/HB distinction was made in all analyses that compared outcomes, for example, cost, site of death, quality of life. The original three-category classification of hospices was retained for analyses that examined possible differences in the organizational changes associated with reimbursement. Although some complexity is added by utilization of both types of hospice classification, we felt that the data would also be richer and more useful.

A Description of the Participating Hospices

We have chosen to describe hospices in terms of their size, staffing pattern (volunteer and paid), use of outside contractors, and the types of criteria they reported using in accepting patients. While there are a host of other factors that may be germane to understanding how hospices function, we feel that these parameters are most relevant to an immediate understanding of the nature of the participating hospices.

The *size* of a hospice program can be defined by a variety of measures, such as the number of paid staff, number of patient admissions, average daily census, and other similar indicators of the volume of resources and activities controlled by the organization. Different measures of size, however, can lead to different conclusions as to which type of hospice is "largest." Size can be measured either by volume of service (number of patients) or capacity to provide care (number of staff). Because one might arrive at different conclusions depending upon the particular definition of "size," we have utilized four measures for each hospice type (see table 2.1). Hospices affiliated with home health agencies appear to be the largest when number of staff is taken as the criterion. We should emphasize, however, that the figures for numbers of staff do not represent full-time equivalents; some hospices, particularly those associated with home health agencies, have only a small core of hospice-trained staff who then draw upon the larger pool of nursing, home health, and homemaker staff in serving patients. Members of this larger pool might then be considered as members of the hospice staff, although they have other responsibilities as well. Once the freestanding and the home health agencies have been grouped together, however, the size differences between hospital-based and home care–based agencies is not as large. Since one of the largest freestanding hospices also had its own inpatient unit, the relative differences were also diminished.

Differentiating between all paid staff and only direct-care staff results in a drop in the average number of staff reported in each type of hospice, although the drop appears proportionally highest in the case of freestanding hospices. This is logical since these agencies require a certain minimal number of admin-

Table 2.1   Alternate Measure of the Size of Participating NHS Hospices

	Hospital Affiliated	Home Health	Freestanding	Hospital Based	Home Care
Average Number of Staff	29.0	45.9	21.2	29.0	32.3
Average Number of Direct-Care Staff	22.2	34.4	9.9	22.0	21.9
Average Number of Patient Admissions per Quarter	29.5	63.5	52.2	36.9	51.4
Average Number of Volunteers Working	19.3	16.9	53.7	26.8	32.1

istrative support staff that might be able to support a larger number of direct-service staff were that necessary to serve a larger volume of patients. Hospices affiliated with existing agencies already have a well-developed administrative structure for functions ranging from accounting to personnel. These functions are "borrowed" from the parent organization, thus reducing the need to develop these functions from scratch.

Based upon the number of patient admissions per quarter, it is clear that the home health agency–based and home-care hospices are the "largest." Even the freestanding hospices, which include several small coordinating groups, on average admit more patients onto their caseload per month than is the case for the average hospital-based hospice. The availability of inpatient beds may affect the perceived volume of patients that can be served. With a fixed number of beds, a hospital-based hospice may be unwilling to admit too many more patients into its program than can be accommodated in its inpatient unit. On the other hand, the home health agency hospice can expand its service much more rapidly merely by drawing upon staff from other parts of the agency. Additionally, at a time when fewer patients are being admitted, the agency is able to contract the number of staff serving hospice patients by transferring them to other services within the agency. While the freestanding agencies do not have that kind of flexibility, they are able to expand and contract to some extent by using contractors, such as visiting nurse and other community nursing agencies, to serve their patients' needs at home.

Not only is the average home-oriented type of hospice larger than the hospital-based variety, but the proportion of small and large hospices is very different as well. A "small" hospice was defined as one that admitted only a dozen or more patients per quarter. None of the home health agencies and only one of the freestanding hospices were that small, but 22 percent of the hospital-affiliated hospices met that criterion. On the other hand, only about 5 percent of the hospital-affiliated but over 55 percent and 41 percent of home health and freestanding hospices were "large" (admitting more than fifty patients per quarter). (See figure 2.1).

The final parameter of size that also reflects the staffing pattern of the hospice relates to the number of volunteers the hospice uses. As can be seen in table 2.1, freestanding hospices are the big users of volunteers. The average number of volunteers working refers to the number of unpaid staff who actually volunteered during a given month and not the number of volunteers available to the hospice as a labor pool at any given time. This latter figure is almost invariably larger than the number of volunteers working. As will be seen in chapter 10, the pattern of use of volunteers also differs across the different types of hospices, with freestanding hospices willing to use volunteers in administrative as well as direct-care types of activities.

The largest group of *staff* in a hospice is its nurses. Based upon an anonymous staff survey of paid and unpaid staff working in participating National

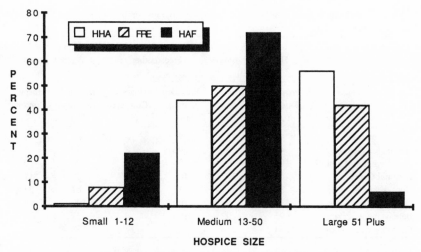

Figure 2.1   Quarterly Admissions by Hospice Type

Hospice Study hospices undertaken in 1981, we found that nearly half (47.7 percent) of all paid hospice staff were nurses. This proportion was somewhat higher in the two traditional types of health-care organizations, i.e., hospital-affiliated and home health agency hospices. The next highest group of survey respondents (16.4 percent) employed by hospices was the health aides, working either on inpatient or home-care units. Other direct-care staff such as social workers, bereavement counselors, and occupational, physical, and nutritional therapists accounted for 13.7 percent of staff, while administrative staff constituted about 20 percent of staff between administrators (who might also be clinically involved in the program) and secretarial and clerical staff. Survey results indicated that approximately one volunteer in eight was a professional. Since women dominate the caregiving professions, it is not surprising that less than 10 percent of paid hospice staff were male. On the other hand, nearly 30 percent of paid staff had family incomes of greater than $30,000 in 1981 dollars. Since hospice staff are not generally paid that well, it is likely that a substantial proportion of the staff is married with working spouses.

One other mechanism serving patients' needs was to contract for or arrange for additional services by relying upon other agencies, generally home health or homemaker groups. Based upon a detailed survey and site visit discussions with participating hospice agency directors, we determined whether hospices contracted for any of a series of different services generally considered to be part of the core of hospice services. Table 2.2 presents the percentage of hospices of each type that reported that they contracted for a range of different services. Since a hospice can either provide a service directly through its own staff or contract for that same service, we have differentiated and analyzed these

Table 2.2   National Hospice Study–Selected Hospice Program Services by Mode of Provision and Organizational Type

	Hospital Based (N = 19)		Freestanding (N = 12)		Home Health Agency Based (N = 9)	
	Provided Directly (%)	Hospice Contract (%)	Provided Directly (%)	Hospice Contract (%)	Provided Directly (%)	Hospice Contract (%)
Home Nursing	47	53	92	8	89	11
Home Health Aide	47	53	92	8	89	11
Pain/Symptom Control	100	0	100	0	100	0
Personal Care	63	37	100	0	89	11
Housekeeping	32	58	42	33	67	33
Family Counseling	90	0	100	0	100	0
Bereavement Service	95	0	100	0	89	0
Financial Counseling	74	21	75	17	78	11

alternatives. As can be seen, hospital-affiliated hospices are most likely to contract for nursing and aides services and least likely to provide them independently.

Inpatient services, not shown here, represent a different problem altogether, since home-care agencies under the demonstration had the opportunity to make contractual arrangements but generally chose not to do so. Consequently, when circumstances required it, home-care hospices' patients were admitted to the hospital to which their physician had privileges, although hospices did reportedly make an effort to consolidate their patients into a small number of hospitals with which the hospice staff could work to assure continuity of their palliative treatment program. As will be seen in chapters 4 and 5, patients served in home-care settings used inpatient settings much more sparingly than those in hospital-based hospices. This reduced rate of use may have emerged from the fact that inpatient services are less available for home-care hospices.

The issue of clinical control is crucial if the hospice philosophy is to influence the actual pattern of care. It cannot be assumed that all hospices have equal control. Hospices that must contract for clinical services may lose some of their enthusiasm and knowledge that their own staff display in providing care when staff of another agency, even one oriented to hospice goals, provide the care. Perhaps even more complicated is the situation in which a home-care patient requires inpatient admission, but that occurs in a hospital without any emphasis on a palliative approach to care. Under these circumstances, the home-care hospice may lose all clinical control of the types of care provided the patient, since the standard operating procedures of the hospital apply rather than the much more restricted clinical approach of an inpatient hospice. Both hospital-based and home-care hospices faced challenges to their ability to exercise clinical control and assure continuity of care. Only the few freestanding hospices that had their own inpatient units were in a position to exercise clear control of care on both an inpatient and outpatient basis.

Hospice care is traditionally associated with treatment of the terminally ill cancer patient. Clearly, however, not all terminal patients have diagnoses of cancer. Nonetheless, cancer has historically been linked to the hospice movement because the image of terminal cancer evokes such strong reactions from the public and because its course is fairly predictable. The predominance of cancer as a diagnostic class is particularly evident in the literature, which invariably refers to cancer patients when nursing or other patient-care issues are discussed. The vast majority of patients served by both the demonstration and nondemonstration hospices had diagnoses of cancer, although the NHS demonstration project did not limit eligibility to cancer patients. This strongly suggests that not only do hospices orient their selection of patients to those with cancer, but also the public views hospice care as a service devoted to the care of the terminally ill cancer patient.

Another feature of hospices that is traditional is the focus on the patient and family as the unit of care. Having a family member be a recipient of care as well as one who provides help for the patient at home then becomes an important aspect of who a hospice patient is and can be. For patients without family, the hospice model is bereft of a family member to serve, and such patients will be cared for at home only with considerable difficulty and expense. The presence of a primary care person (PCP), therefore, is a key to the determination of who is regarded as an appropriate hospice patient. Having a PCP was a requirement for Medicare patients in the demonstration hospices; however, there was no precise stipulation as to who could be a PCP. Consequently, in some instances, there were nonfamily PCPs. Nonetheless, the hospices did not have to limit themselves to patients with PCPs for non-Medicare patients or as a matter of policy for the agency. However, well over half of the hospices had a requirement that a patient had to have a PCP—and for freestanding hospices, 84 percent required a PCP. This high level of PCP requirement among freestanding hospices could reflect their reliance upon family members to provide care at home, or it could be an expression of the program's integrity insofar as serving both the patient and family as a part of the hospice intervention is concerned. As will be seen in chapters throughout this volume, the availability of family support makes an important difference in the amount and type of care provided patients, regardless of whether they are served in a hospital or a home-based hospice program.

A Description of the Hospice Patients in the National Hospice Study

During the course of the NHS, 13,374 patients were admitted to participating demonstration and nondemonstration hospices. Data are available regarding all demonstration hospice admissions over a twenty-four-month period and for an

Table 2.3   Demographic and Functional Characteristics of Sample 1: Hospice Patients' Admissions by Demonstration Status and Hospice Type

	All Demonstration Patients		All Nondemonstration Patients		Total	
	% HC (N = 7161)	% HB (N = 4298)	% HC (N = 793)	% HB (N = 1122)	% HC (N = 7954)	% HB (N = 5420)
Age						
21–44	5.7	4.6	8.3	3.7	6.0	4.4
45–54	9.2	9.2	11.9	8.9	9.5	9.1
55–64	21.4	21.5	21.2	18.6	21.4	20.9
65–74	34.8	35.5	32.3	31.5	34.6	34.7
75+	28.9	29.1	26.3	37.3	28.6	30.8
Sex						
Female	52.4	51.9	56.4	55.7	53.2	52.1
Male	47.6	48.1	43.6	44.3	46.8	47.9
Marital Status						
Married	61.8	56.1	62.1	52.7	61.8	55.4
Not Married	38.2	43.9	37.9	47.3	38.2	44.6
Patient Living Arrangement						
Alone	8.8	18.0	15.7	21.5	9.4	18.8
With Spouse	38.6	40.4	55.5	50.9	40.3	42.8
With Other	52.6	41.6	28.9	27.5	50.3	38.4
Relationship of PCP to Patient						
Spouse	55.9	52.5	58.5	48.4	56.1	51.7
Child	25.4	28.6	23.2	32.8	25.2	29.5
Other	18.7	18.8	18.3	18.8	18.8	18.8
Is PCP Currently Employed?						
No	67.8	59.8	58.5	47.9	67.1	57.2
Yes	32.2	40.2	41.5	52.1	32.9	42.8
Patient's Ability to Walk						
Can Do Alone	25.5	16.8	39.3	16.8	26.8	16.8
Needs Assistance	45.3	40.6	38.6	39.4	44.7	40.4
Unable to Do	29.2	42.5	22.0	43.8	28.5	42.7
Patient Continence						
Continent	42.6	25.6	42.5	25.6	42.6	25.6
Partially Continent	43.1	48.0	40.5	51.8	42.9	48.6
Incontinent	14.2	26.5	17.1	22.6	14.5	25.9
Patient's Ability to Dress Self						
Can Do Alone	16.3	11.9	33.7	13.8	17.8	12.2
Needs Assistance	46.4	42.2	45.7	35.7	46.4	41.2
Unable to Do	37.2	45.9	20.6	50.6	35.8	46.6

average of twelve months for nondemonstration hospices. Table 2.3 summarizes the demographic, functional, and support characteristics of demonstration and nondemonstration patients, broken down by the type of hospice to which they were admitted. In view of the number of patients in each of the groups, no statistically based comparisons were made since "small" differences may reach statistical significance. Since these data represent the population of admissions, the percentages reported reflect the actual distribution of the patient characteristics in the population. Comparisons by demonstration status or hospice type with differences over five percentage points can generally be assumed to be statistically significant.

The age distribution of hospice patients is skewed toward those of advanced years, although less so than one finds with a long-term-care nursing home population (where the largest age cluster is comprised of those seventy-five or older). With the exception of the nondemonstration hospice hospital-based group, all other settings had less than 30 percent of the population seventy-five years of age or older. Another major difference from the traditional long-term-care population is the fact that almost half of all admissions are males and that nearly 60 percent are married. Home-care hospice patients are even more likely to be married and are also less likely to be living alone. Indeed, the largest differences between home-care (HC) and hospital-based (HB) settings are reflected in the patients' living arrangements and their functional status on admission to hospice care. Not only are a higher percentage of HB patients living alone, but HB PCPs are also more likely to be employed, meaning that the amount of time available to provide direct care to the patient at home is greatly reduced.

With respect to differences in functional status, HB patients either in demonstration or nondemonstration settings are more likely to be unable to walk than are HC patients and are more likely to be incontinent at the time of hospice admission. Thus, based upon these data, HB patients appear to have less social support than HC patients and seem to be more "needy" at the time of admission. Despite these observed differences, however, the two groups of patients are not drawn from totally different populations of patients since the differences that we see are not that large, only in the 5 percent to 10 percent range.

Another insight into the differences in the patients served by hospice and nonhospice settings is their length of stay and discharge disposition from hospice care. As can be seen in table 2.4, the vast majority of patients served in either form of hospice care are dead upon discharge. The only exception to that is the nondemonstration home-care hospice group, in which only 63.6 percent of patients are dead at the time of discharge. This is largely attributable to several sites in which the data-collection process was halted without our being able to ascertain the discharge disposition of recent admissions. Indeed, among those patients not dead upon discharge, most stayed in hospices for a long time, and we were not able to continue to monitor their discharge disposition once the project data-collection effort had ceased. However, among the remaining non-discharged patients, regardless of the setting, some small number of patients went into remission, some were discharged due to personal choices, and in some cases, patients were discharged if they had to be admitted to nursing homes. It is not known exactly what proportion of patients fits into this group, but we estimate that it is less than 1 percent of all admissions.

Examining the length-of-stay distribution across the two types of hospices

Table 2.4   Discharge Disposition of Sample 1: All Hospice Patient Admissions by Demonstration and Hospice Type

	All Demonstration Patients		All Nondemonstration Patients		Total	
	% HC (N = 7161)	% HB (N = 4298)	% HC (N = 793)	% HB (N = 1122)	% HC (N = 7954)	% HB (N = 5420)
Reason for Discharge						
Death	84.1	88.8	63.6	85.7	82.0	88.1
Patient Withdrew	3.1	1.3	10.2	0.9	3.8	1.2
PCP Withdrew	0.7	0.2	0.5	0.0	0.6	0.1
Unknown and All Other	9.0	6.9	7.8	10.3	8.7	7.7
Patient Not Discharged	3.1	2.9	17.8	3.1	4.8	2.9
Site of Death						
Home	55.2	21.0	31.4	12.1	53.1	19.1
Inpatient Hospice Unit	·0.5	64.8	2.5	71.5	0.7	66.3
Acute Hospital	20.4	5.3	30.9	2.9	21.3	4.8
Other Inpatient Unit	11.0	2.6	4.0	1.5	10.4	2.3
Other/Unknown	9.8	3.4	13.4	8.8	9.7	4.6
Patient Not Discharged	3.1	2.9	17.8	3.1	4.8	2.9
Length of Stay (days) for Patients Known to be Discharged						
0–7	16.6	25.5	13.3	35.1	16.3	27.4
8–21	21.6	23.0	22.5	25.4	21.7	23.5
22–35	14.3	12.4	12.7	11.9	14.1	12.3
36–56	14.2	13.2	12.2	10.3	14.0	12.6
57–84	10.7	9.0	13.9	7.3	11.0	8.7
85–179	15.6	11.5	14.9	6.7	15.5	10.5
180–210	2.0	1.3	2.8	1.4	2.1	1.3
211+	5.0	4.1	7.8	1.9	5.2	3.7
Percentage of Nondischarged Patients in Each Length-of-Stay Group						
0–84	None	None	None	None	None	None
85–179	1.5	1.3	2.1	0.0	1.6	1.1
180–210	26.7	32.6	18.2	16.7	25.2	27.9
211+	45.2	50.6	73.2	60.4	55.3	52.8

reveals that patients admitted to hospital-based settings are more likely to be discharged within seven days of admission (this almost invariably is due to death). Between 25 and 35 percent of HB patients are served for a week or less, in contrast to about 16 percent of HC admissions. This finding is consistent with the fact that HB patients appear to enter hospice care in a more functionally debilitated condition. Overall, well over half of all hospice admissions are discharged within thirty-five days of admission, emphasizing the short-term nature of the hospice intervention.

One final observation with respect to the characteristics of hospice patients served in both types of hospices relates to the differences in discharge disposition among those patients discharged dead. Among demonstration home-care hospice patients, over 50 percent die at home, while only 21 percent of HB patients die at home. The nondemonstration hospice differences are somewhat smaller, but HC patients are still twice as likely to die at home than are HB nondemonstration patients, without even taking into consideration that discharge disposition data are not available for many nondemonstration HC patients. This issue of the factors associated with where patients die and how families respond to site of death is explored in depth in chapter 8 and has been examined for the population of hospice admissions by Mor and Hiris (1983).

Based upon the differences between the patients admitted to hospital-based and home care–based hospices, questions arise as to (1) whether patients with support from families select or *are selected* into home-care hospices, and (2) whether patients whose families can no longer sustain their rapid functional decline and rising medical-care needs only seek out the hospital-based hospice model of care. We reviewed the list of participating NHS hospices and selected only those hospices located in areas in which the opposite type of hospice also existed and had been operating during the course of our project. Only those HC hospices were included in the analysis if there existed an HB hospice within a relatively short distance from the HC program. The point was to compare the characteristics of patients admitted to each type of hospice who had the potential to choose the other type of hospice.

The results of this analysis (Mor, Wachtel, and Kidder 1985) further emphasized the differences in the types of patients choosing HB versus HC types of hospices. Patients with less-supportive family systems were more likely to be found in HB settings, and they tended to enter hospice care in a more functionally deteriorated condition. The availability of an inpatient setting allows terminal patients without a strong family support system to be served in a hospice. Even if help is available at home, the helpers may have other demands such as employment that make the informal system less resilient and less able to cope with patients' mounting needs. The fact that hospital-based patients have greater nursing-care needs and poorer functioning upon admission may be a reflection of the "breakdown" of the informal caretaking system around the time the decision to forego further active antitumor treatment is made.

The interrelationship between the kinds of patients being served in different settings and how their families assist in and respond to that process is one of the central themes underlying our entire study. Not only do we address the issue of whether hospice care in the United States attains its desired goals of cost-effective humanistic care, but also how the family and the formal health-care system interact to make achieving those goals possible.

3

The Research Design of the
National Hospice Study

VINCENT MOR

This chapter presents the research design of the National Hospice Study. Informed utilization of the findings requires familiarity with the entire data-collection-and-analysis approach. As a complex study undertaken in the "real world," this research effort was subject to its share of constraints and vulnerable to the possibility of both systematic and "accidental" threats to the integrity of the data. In our opinion, the NHS did survive these perils and succeeded in its overall objective of providing a comprehensive, detailed, and dependable assessment of the hospice experiment. Nevertheless, all the information reported in this book should be interpreted within the constraints imposed by the particular research design employed.

Among readers with a keen interest in hospice care, not all will be equally fascinated by a lengthy presentation of the research design. The first section of this chapter, then, offers a capsule summary and then a concise overview. The capsule summary presents the key features of the research design without further elaboration. This summary serves both as an appetizer for those who will be interested in understanding the research design in more detail and as an entrée for those whose appetite is more easily satisfied. The concise overview that follows offers a middle-level description of the NHS design, providing a reasonable basis for understanding the study results presented in chapters 4 through 11. Those with even heartier appetites for methodology are invited to examine the rest of the chapter for detail on site and patient selection, the data-collection process, and, finally, the analytic procedures by which comparisons across patient and facility type were statistically adjusted. A fourth level of research-design detail is also available for those who desire access to the most technical aspects of the study. The reader with a strong technological orienta-

28

tion is referred to the very detailed *Final Report of the National Hospice Study*, available from the National Technical Information Service (NTIS). Since the array of research questions addressed is considerable and a variety of complex statistical models was developed for each, the authors felt that it would not be appropriate to include complete methodological detail in the current volume.

A Capsule Summary

The research methods used in the National Hospice Study essentially compared patients served in hospital-based and home-based hospices with terminal cancer patients receiving care from a variety of conventional (nonhospice) oncological-care settings. We used statistical procedures to adjust for known differences between hospice and nonhospice patients. In general, patient comparisons were made with regard to costs incurred or outcomes experienced over the last weeks and months of life. This focus on time from death controlled for level of disability at the points of comparison. A total of 1,754 patients was included in these analyses, although for comparisons of Medicare costs a total of 3,453 patients was utilized. We also compared changes that occurred in study hospices (N = 40) depending upon whether or not they received special demonstration funding from the Health Care Financing Administration.

A Concise Overview

Sites and Samples

Detailed cost and patient outcome data were assembled on 1,754 hospice and nonhospice patients selected by predetermined criteria from a population of over 12,000 terminal cancer patients who were identified in 40 hospices and 14 conventional oncological-care (CC) settings from October 1980 through March 1983. Additional Medicare billing data pertaining to 3,453 Medicare cancer patients served in hospice and CC settings are also analyzed. Twenty-six of the hospices received special Medicare demonstration waivers allowing payment for normally noncovered services. The nationally distributed study sites were not randomly selected. The demonstration hospices were chosen competitively by the Health Care Financing Administration (HCFA) from a pool of 233 applicants. Because the hospices were selected by HCFA prior to the involvement of the NHS evaluation group, the research design was constrained from the outset. Nondemonstration hospices were selected by the evaluators to resemble demonstration sites organizationally. They were distributed in three areas of the country (Southern California, northern Midwest, and New England).

American hospices vary greatly in organizational structure. After careful review of both structure and behavior, hospices were classified as those with beds (hospital-based, HB) and those without beds (home care–based, HC). Conventional-care settings were selected by the evaluators for their willingness to cooperate and their ability to provide quality oncological care, as judged by the investigators.

The sample considered in chapters 5 through 9 consisted of those Medicare and non-Medicare cancer patients and their families served in HC or HB hospices or in CC settings who consented to participate in a follow-up study. Eligibility for the follow-up study was based upon: (1) cancer confirmed by tissue diagnosis;[1] (2) remote metastasis (except for lung, brain, and pancreatic cancer); (3) presence of a primary care person (PCP), generally a family member in the household (this requirement excluded all nursing home patients); (4) age twenty-one or older;[2] (5) for CC patients only, a Karnofsky Performance Status (KPS) of 50 or less (i.e., requiring assistance in daily activities). These criteria were based upon a review of modal hospice patient characteristics assembled from an analysis of all admissions to demonstration hospices over a four-month period. Over 90 percent had cancer, over 95 percent had a PCP, almost all were over age twenty-one, and over 90 percent required assistance with personal care at the time of hospice admission. As was seen in chapter 2, this profile of hospice patients is consistent with the more than 13,000 hospice patients admitted to participating hospices during our study.

A total of 1,754 patients (833 HC, 624 HB, and 297 CC) was included in the follow-up sample. Trained evaluation staff interviewers assessed patient eligibility from available records. Among those referred to the study in each site who met eligibility criteria, the refusal rate of patients and PCPs (written consent was needed from both) was 3.3 percent, 3.5 percent, and 20.6 percent in HC, HB, and CC settings respectively; dropout among those signing consent forms was 4.4 percent, with no differences among settings. Only patients who died during the study period were included in the final analytic samples since outcomes were assessed in relation to proximity to death.

Data-Gathering Methods

Personal interviews with the patient and PCP were conducted at study entry. A first follow-up contact occurred 7 days later and was repeated every 14 days thereafter until the patient's death. Ninety to 120 days after the patient's death, a bereavement interview was conducted to assess PCP outcomes and to summarize records of utilization of hospital, physician, and home health services, which had been maintained by the PCP while the patient was alive. In addition

---

1. In the following situations, results of tissue biopsy were not required: brain or pancreatic cancer diagnosed through CAT scan; locally advanced head and/or neck cancer presenting visible evidence of lesions; and a diagnosis of leukemia, lymphoma, myeloma, or mesothelioma.

2. We chose to exclude patients under twenty-one years of age, due both to their small number in the hospice population and to avoid issues of parental consent.

to the patient interviews, at each contact the PCP provided data on his or her own condition and attitudes, presented a record of all health services utilized by the patient, and reported on the patient's condition. Information on primary site, histology, metastases, date of disease onset, and prior treatment was obtained from medical records.

Outcome Variables

Based on the National Hospice Organization's statement of hospice goals and principles, we adapted or developed measures to evaluate the impact of the hospice model of care in four areas: pattern of care, patient outcome, family outcome, and cost and utilization. Within each outcome area multiple domains and measures were used. Medical and social service intervention data were obtained from the PCP. Patient and family outcomes were assessed using established scales whenever possible or modifications of established scales developed in collaboration with others in the field. New scales were devised as an outgrowth of the study to address the unique goals of hospice care and to adjust for the rapid decline of the patient population. Patient outcome measures, with the exception of satisfaction with health services, were based upon PCP reports since most of the patients could not be interviewed in the weeks just prior to death. The outcomes measured were overall quality of life, social quality of life, pain and symptoms, and satisfaction with care. Family outcomes focused on the PCP and were measured both prior to and following the patient's death. The family outcomes measured included perceived anxiety and burden while the patient was alive, emotional distress following the patient's death, and morbidity during the bereavement period.

Cost outcomes were based on health service utilization data obtained from the PCP and were checked with Medicare and other reimbursement records whenever feasible. Hospice inpatient and home care–unit cost coefficients were developed using 1982 cost report data compiled either by HCFA or evaluation staff accountants. Cost reports separately allocated all pertinent agency costs to a hospice cost center. All inpatient costs were nationally adjusted based on Medicare hospital reporting data; hospice home-care costs were not nationally adjusted since national standards did not exist. Total costs combine "costs" and "charges" since only charges were available for physician services, drugs, supplies, and equipment purchased at home.

Adjustment for study duration was necessary, given the variability in survival after entry. Since measured patient outcomes were relatively stable until five weeks prior to death, and nearly 20 percent of the patients survived less than two weeks in hospice care, the analyses focused on the period of exposure that potentially affected the largest number of patients: that just prior to death. Patient cost and utilization data were summarized for fixed weekly periods prior to death. Interview data were assigned into these fixed weekly periods. The last measure occurred, on average, seven days before death, and the penultimate measure occurred approximately twenty-one days predeath with no significant differences among settings.[3]

Methods of Analysis

The experiences of hospice and conventional-care patients and their PCPs were not perfectly comparable because, as previously mentioned, the study sites were selected by HCFA on a nonrandom basis. It was necessary, then, to develop multivariate statistical adjustment models. Linear regression (or weighted least squares in the case of total cost measures) and logistic regression models were used, depending on the form of the outcome measure. A different model with distinct independent variables was used for each outcome measure. The independent variables described the characteristics of the subjects at the point of study entry and were selected by analysts based on their known or presumed relationship to the outcome in question. Separate equations were formed for the HC, HB, and CC samples, assuming complete interaction between setting and the independent variables.[4]

Sensitivity analyses were carried out for particular subgroups of patients, depending upon the outcome dimension. For example, patient quality of life analyses tested differences in the estimated outcome variable specifically for patients having high or low values of the outcome at study entry; cost analyses tested specifically for non-Medicare effects because of the salience of payment availability. Given the regression point estimate approach used, all outcome results presented here have been adjusted for differences in the comparison samples. Statistical significance is noted in the text when it reached the $p < .05$ level using a two-tailed test.

The analytic approach used to compare the Medicare costs incurred by terminal cancer patients in the last year of life is identical to that described above. However, the sample analyzed and the data available differed. The sample was based upon Medicare beneficiaries with a cancer diagnosis who died. Hospice patients were only from demonstration sites, while CC patients included Medicare cases identified from the records of participating sites in addition to CC follow-up sample patients. Cost and utilization data were derived from Medicare bill summaries as well as from a detailed billing system established to document services provided to demonstration hospice patients. These billing data

---

3. We tested the differences in patient survival in the study groups controlling for disease, performance status, and selected symptoms, as well as the amount of time patients were able to be followed, and found no statistically significant differences. While our study design is not amenable to testing for survival, these results parallel those Kane and his colleagues (1984) observed in a single-site, randomized clinical trial of hospice care.

4. Detailed equations are available from the authors or in our final report filed with the National Technical Information Service.

provide a complete picture of all Medicare-covered inpatient and home-care services but exclude physician care.

Analyses of the response of demonstration hospices to the availability of reimbursement from Medicare were based upon longitudinal comparisons of demonstration and nondemonstration hospice organizations. Recognizing that the demonstration and nondemonstration hospices were not randomly selected from the outset, we examined the rate at which they appeared to have changed or not changed over the course of the demonstration in terms of a broad series of theoretically relevant variables. Thus, changes in the use of volunteers in direct-care roles as well as changes in the size of the hospice itself were some of the parameters against which demonstration and nondemonstration hospices were compared.

The data used in these comparisons were the outgrowth of multiple interrelated data-collection efforts established at the outset of the study and monitored throughout the course of the study by on-site research field staff. Data gathered included measures of staff salary and turnover (gathered quarterly), monthly data about the numbers of volunteers and how they spent their time volunteering, staff time sheets characterizing the activities of paid and unpaid staff, and aggregated patient data pertaining to all patient admissions during the course of the study. Specific measures of these data were graphically plotted and statistically examined to test the proposition that the rate of change, particularly growth, was greater among demonstration hospices, at least partially as a function of the availability of reimbursement.

The Research Design in Detail

The Selection of Study Sites

In selecting the 26 *demonstration* sites from among the 233 applicant organizations, HCFA used the following criteria:

- comprehensiveness of the proposed hospice intervention.
- soundness and thoroughness of the service plan in the proposal.
- prior existence of the hospice.
- sufficient distribution of the two major hospice types (HB, HC) and representation within each group of agencies exclusively providing hospice care.
- representation of the selected hospices in each of the federal Department of Health and Human Services (DHHS) regions.

Hospice groups submitted proposals in September of 1979, and successful applicants were notified of award within three months. The hospices were located in sixteen states. Twelve were hospital based (HB), and fourteen were home care–based (HC). One of the hospital-based facilities was freestanding (exclusively hospice in orientation).[5] Seven of the home care–based hospices exclusively provided hospice care, while the remaining seven were part of home health agencies.[6] One of the HB hospices did not comply with the terms of the demonstration insofar as they provided no home care. Consequently, it was dropped from all analyses in this volume.

Nondemonstration hospices were selected by the evaluation team. The criteria used were:

- representation of major hospice types.
- similarity to demonstration hospices.
- reasonable proximity to the evaluation project's three regional management centers (southern New England, Minnesota, Southern California).
- sufficiently large patient census to provide patients for evaluation.

Fourteen nondemonstration hospices participated in the study. Eight of these were hospital based, and the remaining six were home care based. None of the hospital-based agencies were exclusively hospices, while four of the HC hospices were exclusively hospices and two were part of existing home health agencies. All had been operational for at least one year prior to their participation in the NHS.

Participating hospice types and the patients they serve were described and compared in chapter 2. In general, demonstration hospices were larger and somewhat more established. There was, however, substantial heterogeneity among participating NHS hospices, both within hospice type and across the demonstration and nondemonstration groups. The variability we observed is characteristic of hospices in the United States, according to leaders in the hospice movement, the National Hospice Organization, and a national survey of hospices conducted by the Joint Commission on the Accreditation of Hospitals (JCAH) (1984).

Given the mode of selection of demonstration sites, it is clear that they do not constitute a random sample. On the other hand, even if HCFA had randomly selected demonstration sites from among all hospices operational at the time, it is not likely that they would have represented the current universe of hospices, given the proliferation of these programs over the past few years. The HCFA-selected demonstration sites and the nondemonstration comparison sites represented the best available estimate of what would constitute hospice care in the United States after the initiation of Medicare coverage.

---

5. A second freestanding hospice classified as HC acquired inpatient beds and hospital licensure in the second year of the demonstration. Throughout this book, patients admitted prior to that time are classified as HC, but patients admitted thereafter are classified as HB.

6. One HC demonstration site (a home health agency) in actuality represents five distinct visiting nurses agencies that are geographically adjacent. Throughout this book they are considered as a single entity (focusing upon the largest of the five) since that is how they applied.

From the perspective of the evaluation, conventional care is essentially all health care received by terminal patients not enrolled in a hospice program. With the growth of the hospice movement, it has become increasingly difficult to locate areas that do not have active hospice programs operating either independently or in conjunction with existing hospital and/or home health agency providers. The NHS chose to locate "access points" to identify patients otherwise similar to those receiving hospice care but who were not receiving it. Conventional care (CC) usually involves multiple programs and sites and frequently several physicians. Patients identified while receiving outpatient services in one setting, for example, may be hospitalized elsewhere.

The NHS selected conventional-care sites representing, in the opinion of knowledgeable area physicians, "good" oncological care. It was reasoned that since HCFA selected what were considered the "best" hospices, qualitative opinion should also be considered in selecting CC comparison sites. Thus, conventional-care sites were selected using the following criteria:

- ease of access in identification of potential patients (for example, cancer registry or up-to-date record-keeping systems).
- conditions conducive to follow-up (for example, integrated medical records and access to billing information).
- willingness of key physicians and nurses to participate in facilitating implementation.
- proximity to regional management centers.

Twelve sites participated in the primary study, supplemented by additional conventional-care settings used to access patients' records and billing data. All CC sites were hospitals or outpatient departments of hospitals. Approval was obtained from the hospitals' institutional review boards, which reviewed the overall study protocol. In each setting, a principal physician (generally an oncologist) was involved in recruiting patients into the study and facilitating the collaboration of other physicians.

Study Patient Samples

Two distinct but overlapping patient samples were used to address the central research questions:

Medicare cancer patients include all patients admitted to demonstration hospices between 10/1/80 and 9/30/82 who had a cancer diagnosis and whose discharge from the hospice was due to death. As noted in chapter 2, around 10 percent of hospice admissions were not discharged dead. (For administrative purposes, some HC hospices discharged patients admitted to a hospital or a nursing home, but this was not a common occurrence.) All hospice patients were Medicare eligible, were certified by a physician as having a prognosis of six months or less, and had a primary care person (PCP) available to act as a helper. Presence of cancer was determined on the basis of primary diagnosis recorded by field staff abstracting hospice patient records.

This sample also includes CC patients found to be Medicare eligible by validating their health insurance claim number with HCFA. They were either identified at CC sites for inclusion in the prospective follow-up sample or were identified by a review of medical records at cooperating CC sites by searching for patients who otherwise fit the sample criteria but who had already died. Thus, all CC patients are known to have died of cancer and to have had a significant other who served as a primary care person.

The *follow-up sample* consists of patients and their families who agreed to participate in a detailed prospective data-collection effort that entailed regular contact with a trained interviewer from the time of hospice admission (or study identification in the case of CC patients) until the patient's death, including an additional bereavement interview with the PCP. Both Medicare and non-Medicare patients with a biopsy-confirmed diagnosis of cancer were included.

Patient Sampling Procedures

In demonstration and nondemonstration hospices, on-site data collectors independently trained and supervised by evaluation staff reviewed intake records and determined the eligibility of each patient admitted. Eligible patients and their PCPs were asked by the data collector to give written consent to participate in the study. If the number of eligible patients admitted exceeded the data collector's caseload capacity at any given time (approximately ten patient/PCP units), the data collector used a table of random numbers to select among eligible cases and only approached those randomly selected.

In conventional-care sites, data collectors reviewed lists of patients under the care of participating physicians or admitted to the oncology unit of cooperating hospitals. The review was performed in conjunction with a designated on-site contact person (generally an oncology nurse-clinician). Permission to contact eligible patients was first obtained from the physician. Then the patient and his or her PCP were approached, and written consent to participate in the study was solicited. Approximately two-thirds of the CC follow-up patients were in an inpatient setting at the time of this initial interview. The remainder were at home or with family.

Ex Post Facto Sample Criteria

Patients spent varying lengths of time in the study, adding a complication to the comparison of outcomes across settings. Some died shortly after the initial interview; others were still alive when the time framework of NHS data gathering had ended. A common frame of reference was needed to compare cost and quality-of-life experiences throughout the entire sample. Since most hospice patients are dead upon discharge from the program, the analytic reference point was determined to be time from death for both hospice and conventional-care patients. This reference point required certain additional adjustments in the composition of the follow-up sample once data collection had ended. Each such ex post facto sample exclusion is described below:

- *Drop-outs* are patients or PCPs who chose to cease study participation; these cases were dropped from analyses because no meaningful "final" measures were available.

- *Patients who did not die* during the data-collection period or who died seven months or more after study entry were excluded from analyses. Ongoing contact with the patient family unit generally stopped at seven months after study entry in order to allow for inclusion of new patients into the study.

- *Conventional-care crossovers* are CC patients who subsequently enrolled in a hospice program. These patients were excluded from the follow-up sample. No such exclusion was necessary for hospice patients who were discharged or who withdrew from the hospice program before their deaths. Once exposed to hospice care, they continued to be considered hospice study sample patients. Thus, such individuals continued to be followed as part of the data-collection effort.

Procedures for Gathering Data on Patients

The data collectors maintained ongoing in-person contact with the patient until her or his death (see figure 3.1).[7] Overlapping sources of data from primary and secondary sources were utilized for each sample, as is summarized in table 3.1. Since the follow-up sample had the most complex and comprehensive data-gathering procedures, the discussion that follows focuses upon the follow-up sample and the procedures used and data available for that group.

At the initial interview contact, the data collector interviewed both the patient and the PCP, inquiring about the patient's condition and recent medical service use, as well as obtaining PCP reports of caretaking behavior and stresses experienced. Additionally, the PCP was given a bill folder and asked to retain any bills pertaining to health services utilized by the patient. Field staff reviewed the service records with patients' PCPs at each contact as a memory aid.

The first follow-up contact occurred seven days after the initial interviews. During this and all subsequent biweekly contacts, field staff attempted in-person interviews with patients and their PCPs. Data gathered from the PCP focused on the patient's condition and quality of life as well as his or her receipt

---

7. The NHS data-collection methodology has been described in detail in David S. Greer et al., 1983, and Vincent Mor, 1984.

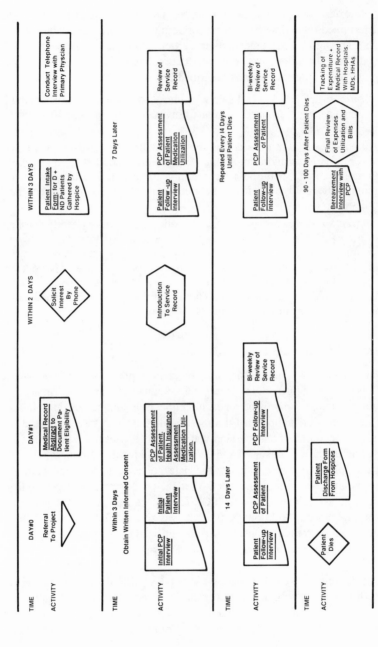

Figure 3.1 Diagram of a Patient/Family Unit's Flow through the Data Gathering System

Table 3.1   NHS Sample and the Types of Data Available for Each

Data Source and Content	Medicare Cancer Patients	Follow-up Sample
Intake Demographics	X	X
HCFA/Office of Direct Reimbursement	X	Medicare
Demonstration Hospice Service Bills		Demonstration Hospice only
Medicare Bill History Bills	X	Medicare only
Medical Record Abstract Disease Stage		X
Successive Patient Interviews (up to 8)		X
Successive PCP Assessments of Patient (up to 8)		X
PCP Interviews (up to 2)		X
Bereavement Interview with PCPs		X
Detailed Patient Service Utilization and Charge Records		X
Medications and Blood Products Use Record		Subsample

of medical and social services. Utilization of all health-care services was recorded. Expenditures for supplies, equipment, and drugs other than those provided by the hospitals or hospices were recorded as out-of-pocket expenses.

A discharge record was completed for *all* hospice and CC patients from all settings, documenting site and date of death. For hospice patients discharged prior to death, reason for discharge was stipulated because hospice follow-up sample patients were tracked even after their discharges.

Detailed information was obtained for a subsample of hospice and CC patients concerning the prescription and consumption of analgesic, antiemetic, and psychotropic medications. If patients were at home, then all drugs prescribed were reviewed by examining the actual bottles with the PCP. If patients were in an inpatient setting, then the medications charts were abstracted. Data on blood product use were also obtained from this sample.

A bereavement interview was conducted with the PCP 90 to 120 days after the patient died. At this time field staff also reviewed with the PCP all service records and bills maintained regarding the patient's utilization of medical services as well as the final reconciliation of out-of-pocket expenditures. Only at this juncture did field staff summarize the total picture of the patient's health service utilization and charge experience during the period of his or her study participation.

Secondary Medicare patient data were obtained from two sources. For demonstration hospice patients, a billing system was specifically established for the project. Demonstration hospices submitted bills to the HCFA Office of Direct Reimbursement (ODR) for any home-care and/or inpatient service provided to participating patients under the demonstration. These ODR bills constituted the basis for examining the utilization patterns and costs of hospice services. HCFA/ODR bills submitted by demonstration hospices were initially screened by claims staff and were then computer processed. Magnetic tapes of these data were periodically relayed to Brown University for incorporation into the overall NHS data base.

The other source of secondary Medicare data was the Medicare Bill History file. This is a summary record of each Medicare beneficiary's inpatient and home health service use. The data were obtained from HCFA Office of Data Management Services (HCFA/ODMS) upon submission of study patients' health insurance claim (HIC) numbers. The summary record on the Bill History file contained all nonhospice bills for a given patient back to 1978. These data were obtained for all Medicare demonstration and conventional-care patients. For demonstration patients, these data represented the nonhospice-provided services received prior to and during patients' stay in the hospice. For CC Medicare patients, they represented all Medicare-covered inpatient and home health services. Not reflected in these data are physician and outpatient clinic services. The follow-up sample, therefore, has more detailed cost and utilization information than does the Medicare sample. However, the greater size of the Medicare sample is a real advantage.

The Analytic Approach to Comparing Patient Outcomes

The principal goal of the research design was to be able to attribute differences in outcomes observed to differences in treatments or programs received. The nonrandom selection of study sites and the design of the hospice demonstration project made it impossible to use the preferred method of randomly allocating patients to experimental and control groups. Another limiting factor in the research design of the NHS was that hospice and nonhospice patients were not drawn from the same population by virtue of their choice of one of the intervention models; they were self-selecting populations. Thus, differences in outcome observed between groups with preexisting differences might have been due to those preexisting differences and not to the treatment intervention. There were differences between HC and HB patients, as well as between hospice and nonhospice patients, that could have confounded the interpretation of differences in observed patient cost or quality-of-life outcomes.

The purpose of this section is to describe the analytic technique used to compare the effect of alternative interventions on the outcomes experienced by patients. The models and procedures were stipulated in advance of our examination of the final data and were aimed at compensating, to the extent possible, for threats to the validity of our findings.

Strategies of Adjustment for Sample Differences

The technique used to adjust for possible differences in the characteristics of the samples exposed to the three interventions was based upon multiple regression models. Two types of models were employed, depending on the kind of outcome variable studied. Continuous-outcome variables assuming values on an interval scale were described by multiple *linear regression* models. Categorical outcomes were described by multivariate multiple *logistic regression* models. In certain cases, analyses were performed using both approaches, specifically where the outcome variable could be viewed as either categorical or interval. In both cases, the models related the observed outcomes to theoretically relevant independent variables.

The four main steps of the analytical strategy were:

- the specification of a linear or logistic regression model relating response (outcome) variables to patient and/or facility characteristics.
- fitting the specified models to the observed data and validating the models.
- the performance of hypothesis tests, specified in advance of inspection of the data, and the evaluation of confidence interval estimates to assess the differences in effects between the alternative interventions (HC, HB, CC).
- systematic use of fitted models to learn which differences in characteristics of patients or facilities are associated with differences in observed effects (referred to elsewhere as sensitivity analysis).

The mathematical models were based upon multiple regression techniques in which independent variables (IVs) described characteristics of patients at study intake and properties of their service patterns. The duration of patients' exposure to the intervention was also used in the models as appropriate. The models assumed interactions between the type of intervention (HC, HB, and CC) and the IVs in the regression equations in terms of how they affected the response variable.

Modeling a response variable Y that assesses the cost of care or quality of life, the *multiple linear regression* equations were of the general form:

$$Y = B_0 + B_1X_1 + B_2X_2 + \cdots + B_pX_p + \text{eps}$$

The subscripted X's denote patient-level independent variables. Three such equations were used: one each for HC hospice patients, HB hospice patients, and CC patients. Separate equations were required because we anticipated interactions between the intervention and other patient-level independent variables. In these models, eps is the random "error" term. We assumed that E (eps) = 0, that is, the variance of eps did not vary as a function of the IVs in the separate equations (though the variance of eps in the hospice equation need not be the same as the variance of eps in the conventional-care equation), and that the error terms associated with separate patients in the samples are stochastically independent random variables. Some hypothesis tests and estimators used were predicated on the assumption that eps is normally distributed. The models were designed with these assumptions in mind. The IVs were selected so that these assumptions would be legitimate, and their validity was tested as the models were fitted to the data.

A different mathematical model complete with IVs was used for each outcome measure across patient cost, quality of life, and PCP outcome domains. Independent variables conceptually related to the outcome measures were identified through discussions with professionals expert in the care of terminal cancer patients, as well as a systematic review of the literature. The array of independent variables from which those included in the models were chosen is large, ranging from standard demographic data to attitudinal information possibly to be related to choice of hospice. Listed below are the domains of independent variables and examples of specific measures.

Patient demographics: age, sex, race, religion, education, income, marital status

Medical factors: cancer site, metastasis sites, stage of disease at diagnosis, comorbid diseases

Family situation: family size, patient and PCP living arrangements, PCP employment status, PCP relationship to patient, family income, other support obligations of PCP, patient's insurance coverage

Prior service utilization: type of prior cancer therapy, prior hospital or institutional service use, prior compliance with physician's orders

Patient/family attitudes: knowledge of diagnosis and prognosis, importance of religion, patient's belief in afterlife, characterization of the aggressiveness of patient's treatment

Extrinsic factors: these include characteristics of the adjacent catchment area (for example, prevalence of hospital beds, home health services, skilled nursing homes), and characteristics of the study site, hospice, or conventional care

Validation of the models relied upon visual methods and objective computational tests. The visual methods served the function of identifying any striking violations of model assumptions that might confound the statistical analyses. Visual methods included normal probability plots of residuals, residual plots against IVs not in the model, and partial regression leverage plots to identify outlier observations. Each has a counterpart in an objective test (Belsley, Kuh, and Welsch 1980). Additionally, computational tests assessed the significance of observed departures from the assumptions. Standard goodness-of-fit tests for the model were carried out provided the assumption of normality was supported (Draper and Smith 1981). Variables not included in the preliminary model that were suspected on the basis of residual analysis to be related to the outcome were tested for significance. The models were then refined by testing the significance of selected interaction effects. Once these procedures had been applied and the linear models accepted, hypotheses about the effects of the alternate interventions were tested.

As a complement to the linear regression approach, *multivariate logistic regression* techniques were used when the outcome variable of interest was categorical in nature (for example, receipt of a given type of service intervention or not). The logistic regression model was based on describing the probabilities for the possible values of the outcome measure Y as functions of patient and/or facility characteristics.

For simplicity, assume Y can assume two values, 0 or 1 (there are natural extensions of the model for multicategory responses). The model expresses the probabilities $P(Y = 0)$ and $P(Y = 1)$ in terms of selected independent variables $X_1 \ldots X_p$. In particular, a relationship of the form:

$$\log \frac{P(Y = 1)}{P(Y = 0)} = B_0 + B_1 X_1 + B_p X_p$$

is assumed, where $B_0, \ldots, B_p$ are model parameters to be estimated (in analogy with the linear regression model described above). As with the linear regression procedure outlined above, a separate equation was developed for each of the comparison groups.

The parameters $B_0, \ldots, B_p$ of the logistic regression models are estimated by the method of maximum likelihood. Our sample sizes for the three settings were adequate for use of theoretical results that describe statistical variability of the parameter estimates. The computable standard errors for the B's allowed us to test hypotheses about the models and to form confidence interval estimates of effects.

Model validation procedures analogous to the ones outlined above for the linear regression approach were carried out for the logistic regression model.

Testing for Effects

The strategy employed for testing whether outcomes experienced by patients treated in HC, HB, and CC settings were significantly different was to estimate the response of the average hospice patient served in a demonstration hospice. This patient prototype was "passed through" each equation to determine the adjusted value of the dependent variable. The null hypothesis tested was: there is no difference in the estimated response of this prototypic patient served in an HC or HB hospice or in a CC setting.

Further, in order to determine whether or not there were structural differences between care settings in the relationship between the IVs and the outcome variable, we tested the null hypothesis that the separate models have common sets of parameters. For the linear model, this was accomplished with the appropriate F-test of the general linear hypothesis (Draper and Smith 1981). For the logistic model, the likelihood ratio test was used (Haberman 1982; Kleinbaum, Kupper, and Morgenstern 1982).

All of the comparative analyses in chapters 4 through 9 clearly distinguish between "unadjusted" descriptive comparisons and those using the multiple regression approach to hypothesis testing described above. A huge number of hypotheses were tested in this study and are reported in succeeding chapters. Part of the reason for this complexity was that many different research questions were asked. Furthermore, as is often the case in relatively unexplored areas of research, we used multiple measures of most patient outcomes ranging from pain to symptoms to service utilization and cost measures. As if this complexity were not enough, we measured most outcomes repeatedly as patients approached death, and each repeated measure of outcome was separately tested using the regression-based approach described earlier. Since different regression equations with different sets of independent variables were developed for each outcome measure, the net result was literally thousands of equations developed, graphically and statistically examined, modified, and then used for hypothesis testing. The results of these analyses form the bulk of the current volume.

Our interpretation of the results of the many hypotheses tested in each outcome domain takes into account the inherent difficulties associated with a study sample comprised of a self-selecting population of subjects. The modeling and statistical manipulations were intended to adjust for inherent differences in the characteristics of hospice and nonhospice patients. Recognizing that unobserved inherent differences may be inferred from observed differences, we can only assume that our models adjusted for these differences as well. If our statistical models did not adequately adjust for differences in the types of patients selecting hospice versus nonhospice care, then our findings can be questioned. Nonetheless, in interpreting the statistical results, we adopted a very conservative stance by accepting a difference as meaningful only if it was consistent and was logically related to other observed differences.

Sources of Procedures for Gathering Data on Hospice Organization

A number of the research questions addressed by the NHS focused on a comparison of changes in demonstration and nondemonstration hospices as well as across the different types of hospices. The central question was how the various types of hospices were likely to respond to the availability of reimbursement. In view of the differences in demonstration and nondemonstration hospices that were documented in chapter 2, our analytic approach relied upon longitudinal data, which made it possible to compare the rates of change of study hospices.

Table 3.2 summarizes the data gathered about study hospices and the frequency with which they were gathered or assembled.

The aggregated patient data provided a vehicle for characterizing the mix of patients served by a hospice and the pattern of discharges, including length of stay, associated with the population of admissions. These data provided the basis for describing shifts in the mix of patients admitted to hospices as well as shifts in the hospice length of stay and the proportion of patients admitted who

Table 3.2   Summary of Hospice Program Data

Data Description	Frequency
Aggregated Patient Intake Cohort Characteristics	Monthly and quarterly
Aggregated Patient Discharge Cohort Characteristics	Monthly and quarterly
Hospice Program Characteristics Form	Once at beginning of study
Staff Salary and Turnover Inventory	Quarterly
Volunteer Statistics	Monthly
Staff Questionnaire	Twice
Staff Time Allocation/Activity Log	Monthly
Facility Cost Reports	Once (nondemonstration) Twice (demonstration)

die at home. These measures provided a gross indicator of changes in a hospice's philosophy or patterns of care.

Staffing data, about salaries, pattern of activities, and the volume and type of volunteer services provided, were also gathered regularly throughout the course of the study. Volunteer data focused on the number of volunteers, the total hours of service provided, and how that time was distributed by direct patient care versus office work. Staff salary and turnover data provided the basis for determining the turnover rate of paid staff serving in direct-care and administrative roles as well as enabled us to contrast the salary levels of staff across the regions of the country. Staff time sheets were aggregated to the organizational level, reflecting the percentage of all paid staff time devoted to direct care versus various types of patient and general administrative time. Staff questionnaires provided the basis for describing shifts in staff skill level as well as perceived level of burden. Finally, hospice cost reports based upon the Medicare approach to cost accounting were routinely completed by demonstration hospices and specially developed based on budgetary and service statistics data for nondemonstration hospices.

Hospice Comparison Analytic Approach

The primary strategy used to compare the differential rates of change of hospices was to graphically display relevant measures from the longitudinal data sources described above. In certain cases, such as shifts in case mix, volunteer use, and staff activity distribution, specific statistical tests of the demonstration and hospice type "effects" were conducted using repeated measures analysis of variance. However, in view of the relatively small number of hospices in the study, such statistical tests were largely confirmatory of trends observed in the graphic displays. The heterogeneity of variance—even within type of hospice—meant that differences had to be very large before a difference

Table 3.3   Analytic Features of Outcome Comparisons in Each Chapter

	Analytic Time Frame	Regression Approach	Special Considerations
Chapter 4: Medicare Costs in Last Year of Life	Medicare costs per month in each month of last year of life	Multiple linear regression with interaction terms	Cost differences "due to hospice" summed across months over last year
Chapter 5: Impact of Hospice in Costs of Last Weeks of Life	Total costs in bi-weekly periods prior to death	Multiple linear regression	Cost differences associated with Medicare status and demonstration hospice also examined
Chapter 6: Comparing Hospice and Non-hospice Interventions	Use of medical and other services in last two biweekly intervals prior to death	Logistic regression subsamples using loglinear analysis	Selected "clinically relevant" profiles contrasted based on cancer status
Chapter 7: Impact on Patient Quality of Life	Outcomes in last three biweekly intervals prior to death	Multiple linear regression and logistic regression	Selected patient reported outcomes examined in reference to point of study entry
Chapter 8: Impact on Site of Death	Cross-sectional where death occurred and from bereavement PCP satisfaction with that outcome	Logistic regression and cross-tabulation	The relationship between site of death and reported satisfaction is also explored
Chapter 9: Impact on PCP and Bereavement Outcomes	Analytic cross-sectional based on the PCP outcomes while patient was alive and 90 to 120 days after death	Multiple linear regression and logistic regression	Pre- and postmortem outcomes examined separately

was detected statistically. For this reason, the statistical basis of the analyses comparing hospices in chapters 10 and 11 is not highlighted. Instead, emphasis is placed upon the graphs and a consistent interpretation of the trends.

Summary

As is apparent, the methodological approach used in the NHS was complex and multifaceted. Wherever we had the leeway, we attempted to control for factors that could have confounded the results of our hypothesis tests. This approach was reflected in site selection and patient selection, as well as in the specification of the statistical adjustment equations. With the exceptions of the analyses of organizational change in chapters 10 and 11, all analyses of costs and outcome used all these approaches to control for the influence of selection bias present in all natural experiments such as this study. Other analytic procedures were also employed in the patient and family analyses of cost and outcome. Depending upon the chapter, these varied from comparing outcomes with reference to time of death to examining only subsets of patients.

Table 3.3 summarizes the analytic features used in chapters 4 through 9 and notes any special considerations or analytic features employed. This synthesis may prove to be useful in reviewing the results of these chapters.

4

The Impact of Hospices
on the Health-Care Costs
of Terminal Cancer Patients

DAVID KIDDER

Overview

Some hospice proponents assert that it is to the advantage of third-party payors to offer hospice benefits because this modality of care is less expensive than the conventional approach to treating the terminally ill patient. Two reasons for hospice savings often are advanced. First, since the hospice model developed in the United States emphasizes care in a home setting, hospice treatment should substitute home care for relatively expensive inpatient care. Second, for those hospice patients who receive inpatient care, hospice treatment is less aggressive than conventional care. Therefore, hospice care should involve less intensive use of expensive ancillary services.

However, there are reasons to believe that, under some conditions, hospices may yield no savings over conventional care. Rather than substitute home care for inpatient services, some hospices might add home services onto the conventional level of inpatient care. Although ancillary utilization and costs may be lower in hospices than in conventional inpatient settings, the emphasis of hospice care on intensive nursing, counseling, and therapy support as part of its routine care could prove more expensive than conventional, routine care.[1]

The following two chapters address the issue of hospice savings. First we explore monthly patterns in inpatient and home-care costs during the last year of life for a sample of Medicare hospice and conventional-care patients. Then we make use of a smaller but more diverse sample of Medicare and non-Medicare patients to describe patterns of hospice costs and savings for other cost compo-

---

1. The NHS methodology treated routine costs in hospice and hospital as a constant.

nents (including physician and out-of-pocket expense). Biweekly data from this smaller sample present a more detailed picture of how costs of care accelerate within the last month of life.

Both analyses generally support the argument that hospice care costs less than conventional care. However, the size, and in fact the existence of savings, varies among patients, depending upon medical and functional condition, personal characteristics, and the availability of home support.

Previous Research

The literature on hospice costs, written over the past few years, has reached a consensus that hospice care costs less than conventional care. However, research findings have been limited by small samples of patients and providers. Frequently cited literature includes the National Cancer Institute Study (Kay 1981), a facility-level cost analysis of three hospices, and several patient-level studies (including Kassakian et al. 1979; Gravely 1980; Creek 1982) on single hospices, each with samples of approximately a hundred patients. Two other studies (Martinson et al. 1978; Bloom and Kissick 1980) focus on small samples limited to patients receiving exclusively home or hospital care. Data reported in these and other studies usually are limited to aggregate statistics without information on the mix of services or composition of costs. A recent New York State Department of Health study (1982) of the utilization and cost experience of patients in their hospice demonstration is an exception.

Factors That Affect Hospice Savings

The existence of hospice savings depends on the particular characteristics of hospice organizations and on the patients who elect to receive hospice care. Among NHS sites, the distinction between home-care hospices that did not directly provide inpatient beds and hospital-based, or bedded, hospices was an important determinant of cost and utilization patterns. Although some of the savings attributable to hospice care depend on the type of hospice a patient elects, there are other important issues related to patient characteristics that the methodology must address.

- *Costs per day and thus relative hospice savings vary with the length of time before death over which costs are measured.* Since it was impossible to determine reference points for conventional-care patients that corresponded to hospice entry, there was no way to compare hospice and conventional-care costs by length of stay. Instead, these analyses compared hospice cost with conventional-care cost over "similar" fixed time periods before death.

- *Patient mix (age, sex, cancer diagnosis) affects hospice costs.* Thus estimates of hospice savings were also adjusted for patient mix.

- *Costs may be affected by prior health-services utilization.* In addition, the decision to enter a hospice may not conform exactly to the date of hospice enrollment. Cost reductions (or increases) could occur prior to the measured date of hospice entry if patients decide to enter a hospice and anticipate entry by changing their levels of utilization. Thus, the NHS methodology estimated relative savings for hospice patients with varying lengths of hospice stay adjusting for prior utilization, measured in the year before the last year of life, well before the entry date for most hospice patients.

- *The length of a patient's cancer illness from initial diagnosis to death may affect the level of resource use in or out of hospice care during the last months of life.* It is particularly important to control for length of illness when adjusting utilization and cost in later periods for prior levels of utilization. Length of illness may also interact with costs prior to hospice entry in affecting hospice costs. For example, patients with particularly high inpatient costs during the fourteenth or fifteenth month before death may not be particularly predisposed to high utilization after hospice entry. Instead, these early costs may reflect abnormally high hospitalization levels associated with initial diagnoses made during this early period.

To investigate these issues, the NHS methodology compared the costs of hospice and conventional-care patients with similar age, sex, diagnosis, pre-hospice utilization characteristics, and length of illness during nine time periods over the last 365 days before death. Separate estimates of savings were computed for hospital-based and home-care hospice patients grouped into cohorts defined by when hospice entry occurred relative to death. This methodology produced patient mix–adjusted estimates of relative savings for patients after entry into hospice care.

The hypothesis that hospice care costs less than conventional care is supported if:

- hospice costs are lower than conventional-care costs for comparable patients.

- costs in periods before hospice entry are the same for comparable hospice and conventional-care patients.

If, even *after* adjustment, we find that hospice patients' costs are different from conventional-care costs *before* hospice entry, then the argument that the hospice program reduced costs is weakened. Instead, we must infer that there were systematic differences in the types of NHS patients that chose hospice care over conventional care that the available measures of patient mix did not capture.

In the next section of this chapter, we discuss data sources, the patient samples, cost methodology, and analysis methods. Then we present descriptive statistics that describe hospice costs and compare trends in unadjusted costs and utilization over the last year of life for hospice and conventional-care patients;

interrelationships among costs, cancer type, and length of illness are discussed. Estimates of total cost utilization and hospice saving in the last year are presented, by setting and separate length-of-stay cohorts, fully adjusted for patient mix, prior utilization, and length of illness. Both total and hospice savings are identified by this method.

Methodology

The Terminal Cancer Cost Sample

Cost, utilization, and patient mix data for the Terminal Cancer Cost Sample came from NHS data forms and from Medicare records. The hospice component of the Terminal Cancer Cost Sample included all NHS demonstration Medicare hospice patients with a diagnosis of cancer who were admitted to twenty-five hospices after October 1, 1980.[2] This hospice patient sample (5,295 patients) is a subset of Medicare demonstration hospice patients with complete cost data (6,945 patients). The larger sample included patients with noncancer principal diagnoses as well as patients discharged alive from hospices.

The Terminal Cancer Cost Sample also included two subgroups of conventional-care patients:

- all Medicare patients with diagnoses of cancer who died prior to February 1, 1983, were identified by NHS data collectors as part of the prospective follow-up sample (Sample 4) described in chapter 2.[3]
- Medicare patients were identified retrospectively from participating conventional-care sites; these patients had already died before identification by NHS data collectors but would have been eligible for the study.

The sample actually used in multivariate analyses was somewhat smaller than the entire Terminal Cancer Cost Sample because of missing values in variables used in the statistical adjustment process (age, sex, diagnosis, length of illness, and prehospice costs). However, the sample reduction does not greatly alter the characteristics of hospice or conventional-care samples.

The Calculation of Costs

For this analysis, costs of hospice and conventional care were computed from estimates of national average Medicare costs, set to 1982 levels, rather than the particular cost experience of the sample of NHS sites. This was accomplished

---

2. Patients were excluded from one demonstration hospice that did not comply with the terms of the demonstration in that it provided no home services.

3. As noted earlier, this includes only one-third of the conventional-care Medicare patients in the follow-up sample.

by weighting measures of utilization by national Medicare costs per unit of utilization or by adjusting certain NHS charges, where utilization levels were unavailable. There were exceptions to this rule, however:

- Home-services costs for hospice care were computed by multiplying each patient's hours of home care by the appropriate hospice's average cost per hour of home care. Under the Medicare hospice demonstration, home-care reimbursement covered more than conventional Part A reimbursable services (skilled nursing, therapies, medical supplies, and equipment). Specifically, demonstration sites were also reimbursed for drugs and biologicals and activities of the hospice interdisciplinary team, as well as direct bereavement, social service, nutritional, home respite, and continuous-care services. These comprise on average 18 percent of total reimbursement for home-care cost per day for the demonstration hospices. In this chapter, home-costs estimates included all reimbursable cost items under the demonstration. We feel that this approach captures the difference in intensity of home-care utilization between hospice and conventional care. Had we computed home costs based only on services reimbursable under both systems, estimated hospice savings would have been somewhat larger than shown in this chapter.

- Costs of conventional home care, SNF, and other institutional care were assumed to be equal to charges. The cost of nonhospice physician's and patient's out-of-pocket expenditures were excluded from these cost calculations.

Methods Used to Estimate the Effect of Hospices on Health-Care Costs

Health services provided by hospices are presumed to cost less than conventional-care services. The major problem in testing this presumption is developing a method for comparing similar patients at similar times between hospice and conventional care.

Because preliminary analyses indicate that health-care costs per week for cancer patients are higher for periods close to death than for earlier periods, health-care costs were measured separately for nine periods: each of the last eight months of life and the first four months of the last year of life.

The approach used to estimate the effect of hospices on health-care costs involved comparing the cost per week in each of the intervals before death for patients in hospices with the cost per week in the same intervals for similar conventional-care patients. Groups of hospice and conventional-care patients were compared on such characteristics as age, sex, type of cancer, length of illness, and prior costs (measured by costs during the six months before the last year of life). Remaining differences in relative health costs between hospice and conventional-care patients during hospice intervals were interpreted as the effect of differences in pattern of care.

Results

Costs and Utilization in Hospital-Based and Home-Care Hospices

What Is the Cost of Hospice Care and How Does It Vary by Type of Hospice? The average hospital-based hospice day cost 30 percent more than the average home-care day, $99 versus $76, as table 4.1 shows. However, the percentage difference in cost per patient was smaller than the cost-per-day difference, reflecting a relatively shorter hospital-based hospice length of stay. The total cost per patient of the services provided during the hospice entitlement period was $6,148 per hospital-based hospice patient, 12 percent more than the $5,492 average cost per home-care patient.

These differences extend to extremes of the cost distributions. The home-care cost per patient was skewed toward less costly patients. While 15.6 percent of home-care patients had total costs of $500 or less, this was true only for 9.6 percent of the hospital-based hospice patients. In contrast, 11.6 percent of the home-care patients and 12.2 percent of the hospital-based hospice patients incurred total costs exceeding $12,000.

What Is the Length and Composition of the Hospice Enrollment Period? Home-care patients had a longer length of stay in hospice care than did hospital-based hospice patients, many of whom had stays of less than three weeks. The mean length of stay of home-care patients was 72.1 days, while the mean length of stay of hospital-based hospice patients was 62.2 days. However, most hospice patients received around one month of hospice care. The median length of stay was 37.0 days for home-care patients and 32.0 days for hospital-based hospice patients. (See table 4.2.)

While there were many short-stay hospice patients, some patients remained in hospices for long periods. The percentage of persons with a length of stay

Table 4.1   Cost of Hospice Care (unadjusted for patient mix)

	Home-Care Hospices (N = 4,834 patients in 14 hospices)	Hospital-Based Hospices (N = 2,111 patients in 11 hospices)
Average Cost per Day*	$76	$99
Average Days*	72.1 days	62.2 days
Average Cost per Patient*	$5,492	$6,148

Note: Calculated in 1982 dollars for services provided to patients from date of enrollment to discharge using NHS cost methodology.

*The average cost per day multiplied by the number of days does not yield the average cost per patient due to rounding errors.

Source: Medicare Demonstration Hospice Cost Sample merged HCFA/ODR data base.

Table 4.2   Composition of Hospice Stays: Inpatient Days versus Days at Home
(unadjusted for patient mix)

Setting	Home-Care Hospices (N = 4,834 patients in 14 hospices)	Hospital-Based Hospices (N = 2,111 patients in 11 hospices)
Inpatient (Hospice and Hospital)*		
Mean	7.5 days	17.8 days[†]
Median	0.0	9.0[†]
At Home		
Mean	63.6	43.6
Median	30.0	12.0
Total Hospice Stay		
Mean[‡]	72.1	62.2
Median	37.0	32.0

*Excludes days of stay in miscellaneous inpatient (e.g., SNF) settings.
[†]Includes both hospital and HB hospice inpatient care received by HB patients.
[‡]Includes days of stay in miscellaneous inpatient (e.g., SNF) settings. Mean miscellaneous inpatient days for HC patients was 1.0 days and for HB patients was 0.8 days.
Source: Medicare Demonstration Hospice Cost Sample merged HCFA/ODR data base.

greater than 210 days was 8.2 percent for home care and 6.5 percent for hospital-based hospice patients.

During hospice enrollment, hospital-based hospice patients received more days of inpatient care (17.8 days) than home-care patients (7.5 inpatient days) as shown in table 4.2. Consequently, the percentage of the hospital-based hospice stay in an inpatient setting was nearly three times that of home-care patients (28.6 percent versus 10.4 percent). Once again, median inpatient days in both settings were below mean days, reflecting the effects both of short inpatient stays in each setting and of a significant fraction of hospice patients who did not receive inpatient services.

How Does the Cost of Hospice Care Vary across Types of Patients?   As noted earlier, the mix of patients who used hospice care from site to site varied. To understand how the mix of patients can affect cost, variations in the cost and length of stay in hospices among patients in the research sample were investigated. For this analysis, patients were classified in terms of:

- diagnosis: patients with cancer and noncancer diagnoses.
- living arrangement: patients who lived alone and those who did not live alone.

While few hospice patients have noncancer diagnoses or live alone, there may be relatively more of these persons covered under the Medicare hospice benefit. In the NHS, 6.7 percent of the home-care patients and 5.4 percent of the hospital-based hospice patients had noncancer diagnoses, and 7.4 percent of home-care patients and 14.3 percent of the hospital-based hospice patients lived alone at the time of hospice admission.

Patients with noncancer diagnoses had higher costs than patients with a diagnosis of cancer. For home-care patients, average cost for noncancer patients was $8,302 versus $5,289 for patients with cancer; for hospital-based hospice patients the costs were $6,661 versus $6,118, respectively.

Diagnosis also was related to length of stay in hospice care. Noncancer patients had longer stays in hospice care than cancer patients. The mean length of stay of home-care noncancer patients was over 50 percent greater than the mean length of stay of home-care cancer patients, while the length of stay for hospital-based noncancer hospice patients was 1 percent greater than for cancer patients.

Patients who lived alone had higher costs. The mean total cost for home-care patients living alone was $7,707 versus $5,136 for patients who did not live alone, while for hospital-based hospice patients the costs were $7,712 versus $5,999, respectively.

Hospice and Conventional-Care Costs in the Last Year of Life

Using unadjusted estimates of total cost and its components, we reach the following conclusions in this section:

- On average, conventional-care patients were more costly to care for than hospice patients in the last year of life.

- Home-care hospice patients' costs for the year were over $4,000 lower than conventional-care costs, and hospital-based hospice patients' costs were a little over $1,300 lower. These differences are based upon the entire spectrum of prehospice and hospice care.

- Savings associated *only with the period in hospice care* averaged over $2,000 per patient over the last year of life for home-care patients; the corresponding figure for hospital-based hospice patients was $585.

- Annual costs for patients with long lengths of stay in hospices (more than three or four months) exceeded conventional-care costs disregarding length-of-illness differences.

- Costs per week grew at an increasing rate over the last year of life in all three settings, but conventional-care costs accelerated in the last month of life more rapidly than hospice costs.

- Home-care patients enrolled in hospices for less than one month were less costly to care for both before and after enrollment; for this group in particular, the adjustment process failed to control fully for the effects of selection bias.

- Hospital-based hospice patients with similarly short stays were less costly after hospice enrollment than conventional-care patients during the same period; there was no evidence that they also cost less before hospice.

- Home-care patients with stays over three months saved relative to conventional-care in the last month of life, but also tended to cost more than conventional-care patients just after hospice entry.

- Hospital-based hospice patients with stays over four months showed costs generally equivalent to conventional-care costs in the last month, and costs higher than conventional-care costs during earlier hospice months.

- Principal diagnosis and length of the cancer illness contributed to variations in costs: breast cancer patients were more costly in hospital-based hospices than in conventional care; hospice patients with long cancer illnesses generally had higher costs over the last year of life, whereas length of illness showed no systematic relationship to conventional-care costs.

- The intensity of inpatient care, measured by ancillary costs per day and ancillary costs as a share of total inpatient costs, fell throughout the last year of life for hospice patients; these indicators did not decline measurably for conventional-care patients, however, until the last two months of life.

- The probability that hospital-based hospice and conventional-care patients would use inpatient care rose more rapidly in the last two months of life than it did among home-care hospice patients; however, the probability that patients would use home services rose more rapidly among home-care patients in the last two months than among hospital-based hospice and conventional-care patients.

- Total hours of home care used almost doubled in the last two months of life among home-care hospice patients; increases for hospital-based hospice and conventional-care patients were less dramatic.

- Other costs, such as skilled nursing facility costs, were rarely above 2 percent of total costs in all three settings.

Costs in the Last Year of Life.   During the last year of life, as table 4.3 shows, conventional-care patients were more costly to care for than hospital-based or home-care hospice patients. However, the difference between the average hospital-based hospice and conventional-care patient was small ($2,101), compared to the difference between home care and conventional care ($4,001).

Hospital-based hospice patients' cost advantage is due largely to the influence of individuals who entered hospice care in the last two months of life. Patients who entered hospital-based hospices from three months through a year before death had higher yearly costs than conventional-care patients. Of course, these unadjusted numbers do not indicate whether or not this pattern

Table 4.3   Total Costs per Week in Each Period in the Last Year of Life, by Setting (unadjusted for patient mix)

	Setting		
Days before Death	Home-Care Hospice (N = 3,641)	Hospital-Based Hospice (N = 1,654)	Conventional Care (N = 558)
0–29	$551	$607	$1,482
30–59	433	590	619
60–89	283	345	277
90–119	222	271	167
120–149	194	224	131
150–179	189	204	162
180–209	160	171	137
210–239	135	158	107
240–364	85	94	89

should be attributed to the effect of hospice care or to the patient characteristics of hospital-based hospice patients.

Although longer stays were also associated with higher yearly costs for home-care hospice patients, the average costs of patients with stays of four or fewer months were considerably below conventional-care costs. However, even home-care patients who stayed more than four months were more expensive than the average conventional-care patient. Care of home-care hospice patients remained considerably less expensive than that of hospital-based hospice patients over the last year, even though costs increased the longer the stay in hospice care. For home-care patients who entered hospices between 60 and 365 days before death, savings relative to hospital-based hospice care were larger than savings relative to conventional care. Home-care patients who entered between 60 and 119 days before death were nearly $1,600 less costly than conventional-care patients. For lengths of stay greater than 120 days, home-care patients incurred lower costs than hospital-based hospice patients, but higher costs than conventional-care patients.

Costs accelerated near death in each of the settings, but conventional-care costs grew much more rapidly than hospice costs during the second and last months of life. Although the cost per year of many long-stay patients in both hospice settings exceeded conventional-care costs, home-care hospice patients tended on average to be less costly than hospital-based hospice patients throughout the year. We also note here the higher hospital-based hospice costs, ranging from $10 to $70 per week above conventional care, in the earlier months of the year. These unadjusted differences were small enough to suggest the absence of a statistically meaningful pattern. The fact that clear differences among the three settings emerged within the last two months of life also suggests the conclusion that savings were attributable principally to hospice care rather than to patient characteristics. Estimates adjusted for patient mix and length of stay, shown in figure 4.1, strengthen these conclusions.

The *average* hospice patient, with a length of stay of between thirty and fifty-nine days, was less costly to treat over the last week of life than the average conventional-care patient. Total savings for the average home-care patient equaled $3,752; a total savings *in hospice* of $4,144 was slightly reduced by an excess of $98 *before hospice*. Hospital-based hospice savings of $1,432 were divided between $3,300 of savings *in hospice* but an excess of cost for hospital-based hospice patients of $1,868 *before hospice*. A majority of home-care hospice patients had savings while in hospice relative to conventional care, as figure 4.1 shows. These savings were large and highly significant in the last three months of life. Home-care costs for the third and earlier months were often higher than conventional care. This pattern was particularly evident in and around the intervals during which each cohort entered hospice care.

These data also suggest that the adjustment process did not fully control for preexisting differences between some home-care and conventional-care patients. On the one hand, it appears that home-care patients who entered hospices in the last month were less costly to treat many months before entering the hospice. On the other hand, among longer-stay patients, there was little consistent evidence of savings before or after hospice entry. Long-stay hospice patients typically increased their rates of home and inpatient utilization earlier in the last year of life than conventional-care patients.

For the majority of hospital-based patients who stayed in hospices for two months or less, hospice care proved significantly less costly than conventional care. Costs for hospital-based hospice patients were higher than conventional-care costs in the months just before entry for patients with hospice stays of two months or more. Estimates of costs in the first month show, however, that conventional-care and short-stay hospital-based hospice patients were no different six to seven months before entry.

There is less persuasive evidence of savings after entry for hospital-based hospice patients with lengths of stay longer than four months. In fact, there were large and generally significant excess costs for hospital-based hospice settings up to the last month for patients with stays from four through eight months. As with long-stay home-care patients, the relative costs for hospital-based hospice patients tended to exceed conventional-care costs around the interval of hospice entry. At other times, both during and well before hospice care, hospital-based hospice patients and conventional-care patients were equally costly, which can be seen in the inconsistent patterns of negative and positive savings and the generally low levels of statistical significance.

Our experience suggests that a "pure" measure of the hospice effect on savings will remain elusive, given the nonrandom patient-selection process that characterized the demonstration.

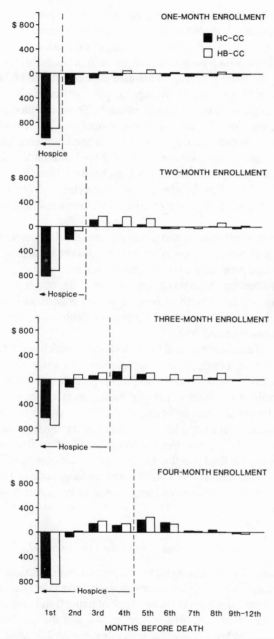

Figure 4.1   Savings Associated with Home-Care and Hospital-Based Hospices in the Last Year of Life, by Length of Enrollment

Costs per Week by Principal Diagnosis and Length of Illness.   In this section, we describe how costs differed within and among the hospice and conventional-care settings by principal diagnosis and length of illness. These descriptive statistics highlight certain patterns not easily seen in the multivariate analyses.

In general, the average conventional-care patient incurred higher costs during the last year of life than the average hospice patient in either setting. An exception occurred with breast cancer patients. Those enrolled in a hospital-based hospice were more costly than conventional-care patients with the same diagnosis. This outcome results in part from relatively higher hospital-based hospice costs early in the last year of life. By the last month of life, conventional-care costs per week were higher than hospital-based hospice costs, at $1,165 compared to $646. Prostate, lung, colorectal, and other cancers cost more for conventional-care patients than in either hospice setting during the last month of life.

Among hospice patients, it was generally true that the longer the terminal illness, the higher were total annual costs. This did not seem to be the case for conventional-care patients. Part of the explanation for the hospice pattern is the association of illness with length of stay. Length of the cancer illness had to be equal to or longer than length of hospice stay. Longer illnesses were often associated with longer hospice stays, which, as we showed above, were associated with increased annual costs.

Costs tended to increase around the period during which patients' conditions were first diagnosed. For the most part, regardless of setting, costs per week in the diagnosis intervals exceeded costs in the preceding intervals by a wide margin. There is also evidence that, for some patients, major cost increases occurred just before the interval of diagnosis. This suggests that cancer might have been detected after a period of hospitalization. For groups diagnosed early in the last year of life, costs dropped immediately after diagnosis and then increased through the final months. Conventional-care costs at diagnosis tended to be higher than hospice costs in the corresponding periods; hospital-based hospice costs in the diagnosis intervals tended to be higher than home-care hospice costs.

The Components of Cost per Week during the Last Year of Life

Inpatient Costs.   Inpatient costs increased for each period as death approached in all three settings, following a pattern that we have seen in total cost per week (fig. 4.2). However, inpatient costs per week of patients in home-care hospices increased by only 4 percent between the second and the last months of life, while hospital-based hospice costs actually dropped by 7 percent. In contrast, conventional-care inpatient costs increased nearly two and one-half times from the second to the last months.

The last two months of life were characterized by changes in the composi-

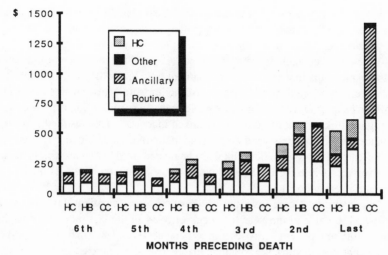

Figure 4.2   Estimated Medicare Costs per Week in Each of the Last Six Months of Life for Terminal Cancer Patients

tion of inpatient costs. In all three settings, ancillary costs declined as a share of total inpatient costs per week from the second to the last months. This change was dramatic for conventional-care patients, whose ancillary costs remained at roughly 50 percent of the total throughout most of the last year of life. Hospice patients' ancillary cost shares dropped steadily from 150 days before death for hospital-based hospice patients and from 120 days for home-care patients. (See table 4.4.)

Table 4.4   Inpatient Days and Ancillary Costs per Inpatient Day in the Last Year of Life for Hospice and Conventional-Care Patients (adjusted for patient mix)

	Setting					
	Home-Care Hospice (N = 2,391)		Hospital-Based Hospice (N = 988)		Conventional Care (N = 407)	
Days before Death	Inpatient Days per Week	Ancillary Cost per Inpatient Day	Inpatient Days per Week	Ancillary Cost per Inpatient Day	Inpatient Days per Week	Ancillary Cost per Inpatient Day
0–29	1.50	$ 61	2.22	$ 37	4.10	$184
30–59	1.26	90	2.02	77	1.76	165
60–89	.81	105	1.05	103	.73	167
90–119	.62	113	.84	127	.55	127
120–149	.54	124	.71	125	.42	132
150–179	.54	133	.60	142	.51	147
180–209	.49	124	.54	117	.46	142
210–239	.39	126	.54	144	.40	116
240–364	.24	125	.32	134	.30	137

Ancillary costs per week are a function of the probability of inpatient use and the intensity of ancillary utilization (ancillary costs per inpatient day, for diagnostic services, pharmaceuticals, and therapies). Some of the decline in hospital-based hospice ancillary costs per week reflected the movement of patients into hospice inpatient settings with relatively low levels of ancillary intensity. However, the probability and intensity of ancillary utilization changed differentially in hospice and conventional-care settings. In hospices, intensity fell even though the likelihood of being hospitalized increased. This resulted from the replacement of aggressive therapy with palliative care. However, conventional-care patients were more likely to be hospitalized and to use costly ancillary services while there. (See chapter 6 for a discussion of the nature of the hospice intervention.)

In conventional care, average ancillary costs per inpatient day rose from below $130 early in the year to a peak of $184 in the last month. Since the probability of inpatient use rose from 59 percent (second month before death) to 97 percent (last month), we conclude that there was an increase in the intensity of ancillary utilization among conventional-care patients.

Hospital-based hospice patients showed a different pattern. The probability of inpatient use jumped from 57 percent to 84 percent, and the costs of ancillary services per inpatient day dropped from $77 to $37. Thus, an increased percentage of patients used inpatient care in the last month and the number of days per patient more than doubled, but the ancillary services intensity of each inpatient day dropped.

Ancillary costs per inpatient day declined between the second and last months for home-care hospice patients, from $90 to $61. However, the probability of inpatient use by home-care patients rose by only 18 percent and the average home-care patient used only .24 more inpatient days per week in the last month than in the previous month. Total costs of home-care hospices did not increase as rapidly as they did in the other two settings because of sizable decreases in ancillary intensity *and* a relatively small increase in inpatient utilization when compared to increases for hospital-based hospice and conventional-care patients.

Home Care and Other Costs.   Throughout the year, and even in the critical last month of life, patients in both hospice settings used at least twice as many hours of home care as did conventional-care patients (table 4.5). Proportions of home care patients that used home services also grew rapidly in the last month (table 4.6). Although probability of home care use grew by around 25 percent for hospital-based hospice and conventional-care patients, it grew by 59 percent for home-care hospice patients.

These figures also dramatize the difference that participation in hospice care made to the use of home services. In contrast to inpatient care, which hospice

Table 4.5   Home Care Hours and Home Costs per Week in the Last Year of Life for Hospice and Conventional-Care Patients (adjusted for patient mix)

	Setting					
	Home-Care Hospice (N = 2,391)		Hospital-Based Hospice (N = 988)		Conventional Care (N = 407)	
Days before Death	Hours per Week	Home-Care Cost per Week	Hours per Week	Home-Care Cost per Week	Hours per Week	Home-Care Cost per Week
0–29	7.4	$195	4.9	$157	.4	$15
30–59	3.8	105	3.0	102	.4	16
60–89	2.2	63	1.8	66	.2	10
90–119	1.4	40	1.3	47	.2	7
120–149	.9	28	.8	28	.2	6
150–179	.6	19	.6	21	.1	4
180–209	.5	14	.5	18	.1	3
210–239	.3	10	.3	11	.1	6
240–364	.2	5	.2	6	.1	4

and conventional-care patients were equally likely to use in the last year of life, hospice patients were more frequent users of home care throughout the year. Among home-care patients, this discrepancy remained clear throughout the nine periods of the year. Among hospital-based patients, the probabilities were similar from the twelfth through the seventh months before death. It is also instructive to note that both prehospice and total probabilities were higher for both types of hospice patient than the corresponding conventional-care probabilities, particularly in the months closer to death.

Utilization of other services (mostly skilled nursing facilities) was modest in all three settings. Other costs rarely exceeded 2 percent of total costs per week in any setting or period: the exception (3 percent of the total) was conventional-care patients in the third month before death.

Components of Hospice Cost Saving for Hospice Patients with Lengths of Stay of Two Months or Less.   We have noted that hospice care was less expensive than conventional care for patients who entered within one month of death. However, we also noted that prehospice costs, particularly for those who entered home-care facilities, were lower than conventional-care costs even after adjustment for patient mix. In this section, we study the effect of hospice care further by showing how the inpatient and home-care components of costs behave for hospice patients with relatively short lengths of stay.

Similar patterns in ancillary costs and home-care services are evident among patients who entered in the last month and the second month before death in both home care and hospital-based hospice. Ancillary costs per inpatient day

Table 4.6   Estimates of the Percent Using Inpatient or Home Care in the Last Year of Life, by Hospice and Conventional-Care Setting (adjusted for patient mix)

	Setting					
	Home-Care Hospice (N = 2,391)		Hospital-Based Hospice (N = 988)		Conventional Care (N = 407)	
Days before Death	Inpatient	Home Care	Inpatient	Home Care	Inpatient	Home Care
0–29	.54	.98	.84	.65	.97	.21
30–59	.45	.62	.57	.51	.59	.17
	(.51)	(.20)	(.54)	(.27)		
60–89	.39	.41	.46	.37	.41	.12
	(.38)	(.15)	(.43)	(.22)		
90–119	.31	.29	.37	.28	.30	.08
	(.30)	(.12)	(.35)	(.17)		
120–149	.27	.21	.31	.22	.24	.07
	(.26)	(.10)	(.29)	(.15)		
150–179	.24	.16	.23	.16	.23	.07
	(.24)	(.09)	(.22)	(.12)		
180–209	.21	.13	.23	.13	.19	.05
	(.20)	(.07)	(.22)	(.10)		
210–239	.19	.11	.20	.11	.18	.05
	(.18)	(.06)	(.19)	(.08)		
240–364	(.33)	(.12)	(.33)	(.11)	(.32)	(.09)
	(.32)	(.09)	(.32)	(.10)		

Note: Percentages not in parentheses are average frequencies for all patients in each time interval. Percentages in parentheses are average frequencies for patients not yet in hospice care.

tended to decline steadily through the last year of life for patients in both cohorts and settings, with a precipitous drop occurring at hospice entry.

For both cohorts, the most significant hospice effect was associated with home services utilization. Hours per week increased by a factor of more than seven times between the second and last months for the cohort entering in the last month and between the third and second months for the cohort entering in the second month. For the latter group, utilization continued to accelerate into the last month, rising from 3.27 hours per week to 11.12 hours per week. These changes were particularly striking because prehospice home care use among home-care hospice patients was not significantly different from the low levels of home services utilization among conventional-care patients.

These data clearly show that home-care hospice savings were a function of declining ancillary intensity and, for some patients, declining numbers of inpatient days per week after entry into hospice care. For the cohort that entered in the last month, these trends were well under way before entry into hospice care. Ancillary costs and inpatient days used by home-care hospice patients were both below conventional-care levels from the third month through the last month of life. Although ancillary costs for the cohort that entered in the second month before death followed the same pattern, a statistically significant "hospice effect" appeared in the last two months of life.

There appears to have been more of a hospice effect on inpatient ancillary costs and utilization among hospital-based hospice patients than among home-care patients. For both cohorts, hospital-based hospice patients' inpatient days per week were about the same as those of patients in conventional care before hospice entry. After entry, even though inpatient days increased more rapidly among hospital-based hospice patients than among corresponding home-care patients, the increase for those hospital-based hospice patients who entered in the last month was below conventional-care levels. The second cohort of both hospice groups showed a decline in inpatient days from the entry interval (the second month) to the last month.

In contrast to the pattern for home-care patients, there is evidence that hospital-based hospice patients used significantly more home care services than conventional-care patients before entry into hospice. This is particularly clear for the group that entered in the last month. Although hospital-based hospice patients' utilization doubled on entry (about half the rate of increase for home-care patients), this represented an increase from a slightly higher base. Once enrolled, hospital-based hospice patients in both cohorts used about two hours per week during the entry interval, compared to three hours per week for home-care patients.

The ambiguity that surrounds the question of how much hospice care contributes to savings is reflected in these figures. Home-care patients in these two length-of-stay cohorts seem to be quite unlike conventional-care patients before hospice entry. They used relatively few inpatient services, compared to those in conventional care, and consumed about the same level of home care services. The principal impact of hospice care for these patients was an increase in home-care utilization and a decline in ancillary intensity. Since utilization of inpatient days did not accelerate into the last months for home-care patients as it did for conventional care, we conclude that home-care hospices provided services that substituted for inpatient care in the last months of life.

In contrast, hospital-based hospice patients resembled conventional-care patients in patterns of inpatient use before hospice entry, even though they were relatively intensive users of home care services. Hospice entry was associated with increasing utilization of inpatient care, declining intensity of ancillary utilization, and increasing use of home care. Instead of substituting for inpatient care, hospital-based hospices added home services to the increasing levels of inpatient care during the last months of life. For some short-stay hospital-based hospice patients, inpatient utilization remained below conventional-care levels, and hospice care was associated with savings. For those with longer stays, inpatient utilization exceeded conventional-care levels toward the end of life, and excess costs replaced savings during the hospice period.

Cumulative Saving Attributable to Hospice Care

By separating prehospice and hospice cost differences, we have seen that savings in hospice differed in size, pattern, and statistical significance, depending upon length of stay. How can we summarize this information and compute a "bottom line" that shows whether hospice care, under the demonstration, did or did not save over conventional care? Figure 4.3 cumulates the net differences, positive and negative, across length-of-stay cohorts in two ways: first, cost differences between hospice and conventional-care patients are shown for each time period, regardless of whether or not the patient was in hospice; second, prehospice cost estimates are subtracted to leave our best estimate of a "hospice only" component.[4] The first measure provides total cost differences associated with hospice *patients* before and during hospice care, after adjusting for patient mix differences. The second measure reflects how much of these differences occurred during hospice care and is therefore a better indicator of hospice savings.

For the last month of life, home-care patients were $3,827 less expensive to care for than conventional-care patients. Adding in all the patient months in the last year increases this difference to $4,288. However, the portion associated with hospice care was only 50 percent in the last month of life (a saving of $1,919), rising slightly to 51 percent when all the years' savings are cumulated ($2,221). This represents a total estimated hospice saving to Medicare for the 3,944 home-care patients of over $5,310,411. Of course, this pattern is conditioned by the particular length-of-stay distribution of hospice patients in the demonstration.

The cost advantage of hospital-based hospice patients followed a different pattern. Rather than increase during the last year of life, the largest cost advantage for hospital-based hospice patients appeared at $3,441, in the last month and declined steadily to $1,362 when cumulated over the entire year. The share of this cost difference attributable to hospice care was smaller for hospital-based than for home-care hospice patients throughout the year. In the last month of life, hospice savings were $1,609, or 47 percent of total savings in that period. After cumulating over the year, hospice savings dropped to $585, representing 43 percent of total savings. Total savings associated with hospital-based hospice care were $477,980.

---

4. It is assumed that one-half of the hospice patients' costs during the interval in which each cohort entered hospice care represents hospice costs and one-half represents prehospice costs. This convention was adopted because problems encountered in dating bills made a precise allocation of costs within a small interval impossible. Our approach recognizes the fact that average lengths of stay in both hospice settings by cohort were located on or near the midpoint of each interval.

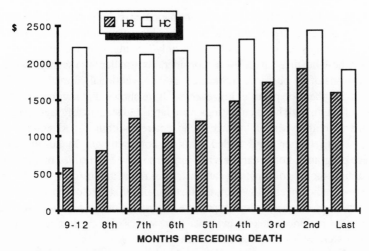

Figure 4.3   Savings Associated with Home-Care and Hospital-Based Hospices Relative to the Costs of Conventional Care in the Last Year of Life

We cannot determine the statistical significance of estimates of hospice-only savings, since these were derived from estimates of total cost differences. However, we observe that estimates of total cost differences associated with hospice care were large for home-care patients, at 15 percent of average total cost of conventional care in the last year. Savings for the *average* home-care patient (thirty to fifty-nine days in hospice) were 28 percent. In contrast, hospital-based hospice care appears to have saved about 4 percent of total conventional-care costs. The average hospital-based hospice patient saved 10 percent.

Conclusion

The evidence reviewed in this chapter strongly supports the hypothesis that home-care hospice patients are less costly to care for than conventional-care patients in the last year of life. We reach the same conclusion, although with less confidence, regarding hospital-based hospice patients. We are confident of these findings, in part because the assumptions behind the cost calculations were conservatively weighted toward relatively higher hospice costs: hospice routine costs were assumed higher than hospital routine costs, and the costs of hospice home care services included expenditures on case management, bereavement counseling, and other services not included in Medicare-reimbursed home care services provided for conventional care.

We have *not,* however, made a strong case for the hypothesis that these savings are effected principally by hospice care. The fact that the largest cohort of home-care patients—those who entered a hospice in the last month of life—were low utilizers of inpatient services relative to conventional-care patients before hospice, even after adjustment for patient mix, indicates that a selection bias was present. The implications of this bias were made clear when we constructed an estimate of total "hospice only" savings over the entire last year of life. These hospice savings were considerably smaller than savings based on comparisons of all hospice, prehospice, and conventional-care costs.

From another perspective, however, we have shown that savings in the last month of life in both hospice settings were large and statistically significant for patients in both types of hospices who entered within 120 days of death. Patients with longer stays added costs in both settings. In hospital-based hospice programs, home-care services appear to have been added on to already substantial amounts of inpatient care instead of replacing institutionalization as in home-care hospices. However, the fact remains that care of most patients in the hospice program was less expensive regardless of the reason. Even with longer stays included, there is evidence that savings over the last year of life in hospices were realized in the demonstration.

Is hospice care a less costly method of care for terminally ill patients, or do hospices simply attract individuals prone to low levels of utilization? Despite the ambiguities we have stressed in our findings, we believe a pure hospice effect operated, though the size of the effect was not measured precisely in this study. Although home-care hospice patients entering in the last month of life were low users of inpatient care before hospice entry, ancillary intensity rose steadily until the month before entry. Intensity then dropped and home-care utilization rose dramatically, while conventional-care patients used more inpatient care. Hospital-based hospice patients who entered in the last month accelerated their inpatient utilization more slowly than did conventional-care patients. Home services utilization increased rapidly for this group, as it did for home-care hospice patients. If, in the future, hospices were to attract patients more prone to use inpatient care, then savings before and during hospice care would be more modest than they were in the demonstration. Hospital discharge practices under the new Medicare Prospective Payment System bear continued scrutiny in this regard. It is possible that payment rates for diagnostically related groups will fail to capture the full costs of treating hospitalized terminally ill patients who have not elected hospice care. Should this prove to be the case, then hospitals may discharge such patients earlier than they would have under the cost-based system of payment. This practice might increase pressure on hospices—and nursing homes—to admit patients not suited for home care.

Nonetheless, we expect that hospices will continue to contain the use of inpatient services and total costs of care near death. In particular, hospices certified by Medicare are constrained by caps on inpatient utilization and total expenditures that should constrain costs by creating additional incentives for home placement.

5

Hospice Services and Cost Savings in the Last Weeks of Life

DAVID KIDDER

In the prior chapter, the emphasis was upon hospice costs to Medicare as well as cancer care costs, inpatient and at home, over the last year of life. Those analyses were particularly relevant for U.S. policy makers in considering the possible increases or decreases in Medicare costs that might arise if hospice care were introduced as a covered benefit. Indeed, we worked closely with the framers of the Medicare hospice regulations that were initially formulated to govern the hospice benefit passed into law as a part of the Tax Equity and Fiscal Responsibility Act of 1982.

Although the analyses presented in the prior chapter certainly do provide a flavor for the differences in the pattern of services received by hospice patients in the two types of hospices and the conventional-care system, certain types of services were excluded, and the important issue of out-of-pocket expenses was not addressed. Additionally, since we have seen that the duration of the hospice exposure associated with the typical hospice patient is relatively short (a median length of stay of around thirty-five days), this chapter focuses on the pattern of services patients receive over the last weeks of life. Thus, while the prior chapter provides the "big picture" so important for policy analysts, the current chapter details the distribution of services within a shorter time frame, comparing the costs incurred and changes in services received among hospice patients in both types of settings as well as in the conventional-care system.

We begin with a description of the pattern of all relevant health-care services received by hospice Medicare and non-Medicare patients in hospital-based hospice and home care–based settings. Comparisons are also made by whether the hospice was a demonstration site or not in order to determine if the availability of additional reimbursed services altered the pattern and costs of services used. A relatively large proportion of hospital-based hospice patients spent virtually all of their hospice stay in an inpatient setting. Therefore, we also describe and contrast those patients and their patterns of service use with those of the remaining patients in order to estimate whether the cost and service-use differences observed between hospital-based and home-care hospices can be attributed to patients who spend all of their time in the inpatient setting. Finally, we present the comparisons of the changes in service-use patterns among hospice and nonhospice patients over the last weeks of life and estimate the cost implications of those differences.

Methods

In this chapter, data collected from 1,621 NHS follow-up sample patients were used to study cost differences (1) between Medicare-eligible and non-Medicare hospice patients, (2) between hospice and conventional care, and (3) between demonstration and nondemonstration hospice sites. For the follow-up sample, we gathered not only costs and utilization reimbursable under Part A of Medicare (inpatient and some home-care costs), but also other costs (fee-for-service physician charges, drug, supply, and equipment expenditures, and other out-of-pocket expenses for health care). These data were obtained from Medicare and non-Medicare patients' primary care persons. The measures of costs and utilization are described below. The outcome variables analyzed, including utilization and cost during short periods prior to death, are also enumerated and discussed. For the purpose of this chapter, hospice patients are grouped by demonstration status (demonstration and nondemonstration), setting (hospital based and home care), and Medicare eligibility (all NHS patients and non-Medicare patients). The analysis concludes with a comparison of costs and utilization in hospice and conventional care.

Measuring Costs

The essential components of the cost methodology described in the prior chapter were applied to patients in the smaller NHS follow-up sample. As discussed in chapters 2 and 3, the follow-up sample included only a subset of all hospice admissions, that is, those with cancer, primary care persons, and those willing to participate in a series of interview contacts.

Even though the definition of total costs in this chapter has been expanded beyond inpatient, skilled nursing facility, and home health, we have not measured the total costs of cancer, or even the less restrictive measure of total costs of terminally ill patients. Studies such as Cancer Care Inc. (1973) and Abt (1975) have identified and tried to measure the value of loss of function, the effects on a family of income loss, and other costs associated with the onset of a life-threatening disease. Some major expenditures, such as changing homes or the capital expense of modifying a home to accommodate a terminally ill patient, may be particularly significant for some families, as Cancer Care Inc. shows. However, these expenses are often difficult to prorate to the task of patient care, particularly if the goal is to determine costs incurred during a relatively short period of time.

Decisions regarding what services and types of expenditures to include in our definition of costs were based both on the feasibility of collecting valid data and on the requirements of the evaluation. Even though loss of expected earnings for cancer patients who die constitutes the largest component of the aggregate social costs of cancer (Rice 1966), there is no reason to believe that choice of hospice care or experience in a hospice will be related to income loss. Loss of income earned by family members who now serve as primary care persons and the value of time spent by family and friends in caring for the patient are topics treated to some extent in chapter 9. Chapter 7 addresses questions of the "psychic costs" of terminal illness associated with lower quality of life, although with no effort to place a dollar value on them.

Most of the variables used to compare costs and utilization among types of hospices, and between hospice and conventional care, were defined as rates per study day,[1] per week, and per patient. Analyses that compared different hospice settings were based on patients' length of stay in hospice care. Contrasts of costs and utilization between hospice and conventional care were based on comparable intervals before death.

Various measures of utilization and cost components were studied to help understand sources of variation in total costs. These were physician services, outpatient services, patient out-of-pocket expenditures (drug, supply, and equipment expenditures) per hospice day, inpatient services, and home care services. Home care services include visits from nurses, home health aides, and other providers such as social workers and physical or inhalation therapists. This component was expressed in terms of visits because this was the common unit for all home care used by NHS patients. The nursing and home health agency (HHA) components were also measured in hours, a better measure of home health-care intensity. For each type of service, measures of costs per day and costs per patient were constructed, as was a measure of the number of units of service per day.

The measure of total cost used to compare hospice-care costs with conventional-care patient costs, based on inpatient and home service, is the sum of each service component's costs or charges during a particular time period. In contrast to the Medicare Bill History data used in chapter 4, data collected from follow-up patients could be accurately allocated to relatively short time periods, since study data collectors validated dates of utilization in relation to patients'

---

1. In discussions of hospice costs, the term *hospice day* is used in place of "study day," which can be applied both to hospice and conventional-care patients in the NHS sample.

entry into the study and their deaths. Therefore, we were able to describe changes in utilization within the last two months of life. Five intervals defined the nine-week period before death:

- 7 to 0 days.
- 21 to 8 days.
- 35 to 22 days.
- 49 to 36 days.
- 63 to 50 days.

In addition to monitoring changes in total costs as patients approached death, various utilization components were also compared over these five intervals. For example, inpatient days per week were contrasted, as were all home-care visits and the number of hours of nursing and home health aide care.

Since a broader range of utilization components was included in our definition of terminal cancer care costs, the Medicare approach to defining costs had to be expanded. To the extent possible, we retained all aspects of the Medicare approach to defining "nationally" adjusted costs for inpatient costs. For non-demonstration hospices we used cost accounting data prepared by our own accountants. Ancillary charges were converted to costs as in chapter 4, except where unavailable, in which case we used average ancillary charges from patients served in similar facilities.

Hospice home-care unit-of-service costs were based upon the average cost of a hospice home visit for the hospice in which the patient was served. An average charge based upon charge data collected by our staff was assigned to all nonhospice patients' home-care visits. Skilled nursing, physician, and outpatient clinic visits were priced as charges obtained by the data collectors. Total out-of-pocket expenditures were recorded separately and accumulated from worksheets maintained by the patient's primary care person. A separate record of expenditures for drugs, supplies, and medical equipment, whether reimbursed or not, was also maintained. There was a relatively short interval between the patient's death and our data collector's visit to the primary care person to conduct a bereavement interview and collate records from the service diary (an average of three and a half months). Therefore, accurate estimates of the amount of final medical bills that were not covered by health insurance were not generally available. Our measure of total out-of-pocket expenditures is thus likely to underestimate true charges, although it is not clear by how much.

Analysis Approach

For the most part in this chapter, NHS measures of cost and utilization are presented as unadjusted sample averages. The final section presents comparisons of hospice and nonhospice patient costs as estimates adjusted for patient differences among hospice types and between hospice and conventional care. The regression methodology used for adjustment is described thoroughly in chapter 3. Although the number of control variables differs, the adjustment models used are structurally identical to models used in chapter 4.

Cost and Utilization Differences by Hospice Type and Medicare Status

Levels of inpatient use for the last sixty-three days of life were substantially higher in hospital-based hospices during all periods than among home-care hospice patients (table 5.1). Even though average inpatient utilization increased nearly threefold during the period from fifty to sixty-three days before death to the last week of life in both settings, inpatient utilization of home-care patients remained about one-half the level shown in the hospital-based hospice settings.

Use of both skilled nursing and home health services increased as home-care hospice patients approached death. Indeed, the average number of visits per week increased by at most half during the last week of life. Combining both types of visits, there were 4.8 visits per week in the penultimate period and 7 in the last week of life. Among hospital-based hospice patients, skilled-nursing use increased slightly in the last week, but home health aide utilization decreased closer to death.

Hospital-based hospice patients apparently used home care, particularly skilled nursing, in addition to increasing levels of inpatient utilization. Utilization rates were nearly the same for both skilled nursing and home health in both hospice settings sixty-three days before death. As patients' medical condition deteriorated, hospital-based hospices appeared to respond by admitting those patients to an inpatient setting (an average of four of the last seven days of life

Table 5.1 NHS Unadjusted Inpatient and Home-Care Utilization Patterns in the Last Sixty-Three Days of Life: Home-Care and Hospital-Based Hospice

Service/Setting	Days before Death				
	7 to 0	21 to 8	35 to 22	49 to 36	63 to 50
Inpatient Days per Week					
Hospice					
Home Care	1.9	1.1	0.8	0.7	0.6
Hospital Based	4.2	2.8	2.2	1.8	1.5
Skilled Nursing Visits per Week					
Hospice					
Home Care	3.7	2.2	1.9	1.8	1.6
Hospital Based	1.9	1.5	1.5	1.5	1.6
Homehealth/Homemaker Visits per Week					
Hospice					
Home Care	3.3	2.6	2.5	2.4	2.2
Hospital Based	1.5	1.5	1.8	1.7	1.8

Table 5.2   Total Costs for Non-Medicare and Medicare Patients
by Hospice Type

	Hospital Based (N = 620)	Home Care (N = 890)
Total Costs per Hospice Day		
Medicare	$ 170	$ 115
Non-Medicare	$ 142	$ 95
Total Costs per Patient		
Medicare	$8,198	$6,259
Non-Medicare	$6,244	$5,108

were spent in an inpatient setting). While home-care patients also spent more days in the hospital in the last week of life than was true in prior weeks, the intensity of home-care services increased considerably, presumably to meet the needs of patients remaining at home.

The different approach hospital and home hospices took to meeting the increasing needs of terminal cancer patients can be seen across a variety of parameters of utilization. The net result of these differences can be seen in table 5.2. As was true of the prior chapter, hospital-based hospice patients incurred higher total costs per day and per stay than was the case for home-care hospice patients.[2] Medicare-eligible home-care hospice patients incurred costs per day that were only two-thirds of their hospital-based hospice counterparts. Differences between non-Medicare-eligible patients served in the two types of hospices were quite comparable to those of Medicare patients, although in both types of hospice settings non-Medicare patients incurred lower costs than did Medicare patients.

Inpatient Utilization

Inpatient care contributes more to the total costs of hospice care than all other components combined. Two parameters of inpatient utilization must be considered: the probability of having an inpatient stay, and the duration of the stay. As can be seen in table 5.3, the proportion of hospital-based hospice patients with any time in an inpatient setting was nearly twice that of the home-care hospice group. Among home-care hospice patients, Medicare patients were less likely than were non-Medicare patients to use an inpatient setting. The increased availability of home care under Medicare, and particularly in the demonstration hospices (which contained the bulk of patients in the sample), suggest that cov-

---

2. There are two reasons why these figures for total hospice costs exceed those presented in chapter 4. First, these include physician, outpatient, and out-of-pocket costs. Second, the average length of stay of follow-up sample members was shorter than all admissions since all follow-up patients had to have died to be in the sample. Consequently, long-stay, nonintensive service users are not included.

Table 5.3   NHS Unadjusted Measures of Hospice Inpatient
Utilization and Costs for Non-Medicare and Medicare Patients

	Hospital Based (N = 523)	Home Care (N = 808)
Percent of Patients Using Inpatient Care		
Medicare	85	44
Non-Medicare	84	55
Inpatient Days as Percent of Hospice Days		
Medicare	40	14
Non-Medicare	33	15
Inpatient Costs per Hospice Day		
Medicare	$110	$43
Non-Medicare	$ 95	$39

erage for home services may have affected the likelihood of using an inpatient setting among patients and families who had already made the decision to have care delivered at home by choosing a home-care hospice.

Hospital-based hospice patients spent a larger proportion of their hospice stay in an inpatient setting than did home-care hospice patients, and in this case, the Medicare–non-Medicare differential is seen among hospital-based hospice patients. Hospital-based hospice patients were both more likely to use an inpatient setting and to stay longer (approximately 23.5 versus 15.9 among hospital-based and home care–based Medicare patients who used inpatient services). It is not surprising, therefore, that inpatient costs per hospice day are more than twice those of home-care hospice patients, whether among Medicare or non-Medicare patients. Thus, at least with respect to inpatient utilization, the pattern of findings seen in chapter 4 also applies to younger, non-Medicare patients having very different insurance coverage.

Institution-Based Patients

It is clear from data gathered in the NHS that many patients served by hospital-based hospice programs never received treatment at home. This is one reason for the substantial difference between home- and hospital-based hospice patients' inpatient utilization. A relatively high proportion of hospital-based hospice patients (29 percent) were in an inpatient setting throughout their stay in hospice care. Responding to the United States' version of the hospice philosophy and seeking a cost-effective model for reimbursing hospices, the Congress included incentives for home care use and penalties for high use of inpatient settings in the hospice provisions of the Tax Equity and Fiscal Responsibility Act of 1982. Whether this was the "correct" mode of treatment for this group or whether it was consistent with the hospice philosophy is not at issue. Indeed, debate continues to rage among proponents of hospice care as to whether a home or an inpatient approach best serves the needs of the patient (Mount 1976; Saunders 1981). At this juncture, it is, however, instructive to characterize those patients who spent all of their time in a hospice in an inpatient setting and to determine whether the differential costs and patterns of inpatient utilization observed between home and hospital hospices are largely attributable to the "institution bound," hospital-based hospice patient.

We compared the characteristics of institution-bound and non–institution-bound hospital-based hospice patients. While similar with respect to age, sex, and cancer type, institution-bound patients were radically different with respect to both length of stay in hospice care as well as the amount of inpatient services used in the two months prior to hospice admission. Institution-bound patients spent about twenty days in the two months prior to hospice admission in a hospital, while the remaining group of hospital-based hospice patients spent only twelve days in the hospital.

Additionally, once admitted to a hospice, institution-bound patients survived less than half as long as did other hospital-based hospice patients, around twenty-five days versus nearly sixty among the remaining group. Consistent with the finding of shorter survival, institution-bound patients were less functionally independent upon admission, and they were somewhat more likely to have lived alone than was the case for the remaining group of hospital-based hospice patients.

As might be expected, the costs per day of the institution-bound patient were considerably higher than for other hospital-based hospice patients. Inpatient costs were over 250 percent higher for institution-bound patients. Even physician costs per hospice day were higher for this group of patients, presumably because they were seen by a physician nearly every day that they were in the inpatient setting.

Based upon anecdotal evidence from the hospice sites, both demonstration and nondemonstration, that served relatively high numbers of these types of patients, it is our impression that many were "internal transfers" from an oncology unit or a regular medical floor of the hospital to which the hospice was attached. This is not the only group, however. Many patients admitted to free-standing hospital-based hospices with their own inpatient unit were also institution bound. These cases included patients admitted from an area not served by the hospice's home-care program as well as patients transferred into the hospice from nearby medical centers. In either case, these patients were often admitted with the knowledge that they would not return home. This use of the hospice is reminiscent of the hospice in the United Kingdom as well as in Canada. How, and indeed whether, it should be incorporated into the legislative and regulatory confines of a hospice reimbursement system will continue to be an important issue in the future.

It is interesting to note that even once the institution-bound patients have been eliminated from consideration, the level of inpatient service use of hospital-based hospice patients remains significantly higher than that of home-care patients. Total inpatient days of the remaining hospital-based hospice patients averaged around fifteen days, while home-care patients averaged only around seven days. This translates into an inpatient cost per hospice day of around $70 for the hospital-based hospice patients and around $42 for home-care patients. Thus, while eliminating the institution-bound patients from the comparisons does reduce the level of differences observed, it by no means eliminates them.

Home-Care Utilization

A goal of many hospice programs across the country is to enable patients to choose whether death should occur at home or in an inpatient setting. Home-care utilization, like inpatient-care use, varied considerably among hospice settings. As can be seen in table 5.4, almost all home-care patients, regardless of payor (Medicare status), used home care, whereas only about two-thirds of hospital-based hospice patients received home-care services. Medicare patients appear to have received more visits per hospice day than was the case for non-Medicare patients. This difference due to payor type operates across both types of hospices. The effects of these differences can also be seen in the cost per hospice day attributable to home-care services. For both types of hospices, Medicare patients' costs are about $14 per day higher than those for non-Medicare patients. Since the majority of all patients are from demonstration hospices and the majority of them are Medicare beneficiaries, it is reasonable to assume that the availability of Medicare benefits, particularly among demonstration patients, contributed to the higher use of these services among Medicare patients. In a later section of this chapter we will examine the apparent contribution of demonstration status to the observed differential in home-care use in order to determine whether it was Medicare or the special services available under the

Table 5.4   NHS Unadjusted Measures of Hospice Home-Care Utilization and Costs for Non-Medicare and Medicare Patients

	Hospital Based (N = 523)	Home Care (N = 808)
Percent of Patients Using Home Care		
Medicare	65	100
Non-Medicare	63	99
Home Care Visits per Hospice Day		
Medicare	0.52	0.79
Non-Medicare	0.40	0.53
Home Care Costs per Hospice Day		
Medicare	$49	$57
Non-Medicare	$35	$43

demonstration that contributed to higher daily home-care costs among Medicare patients.

Physician and Outpatient Services

We gathered patient-specific data about physician services provided by physicians who billed separately for services delivered in inpatient or office settings. Services provided through outpatient clinics included physician and nonphysician components, although it was clear that many hospice patients—particularly those in home-care settings—received physician care in this manner (table 5.5). Physician and outpatient services combined constituted the largest part of health-care costs other than inpatient and home care for hospice patients. Adding physician and outpatient costs per day and then dividing them into total costs per day (see table 5.2) reveals that, depending upon hospice type and payor source, physician services account for between 5 percent and 10 percent of total daily direct hospice costs.

As can be seen in table 5.5, the home-care patients, regardless of payor source, are most likely to have used outpatient clinics, presumably for palliative treatment or follow-up observation after active treatment had ceased. Physician services were reported by about three-quarters of all hospital and home-care Medicare hospice patients. Non-Medicare patients in hospital-based hospice settings were somewhat more likely than their home-care counterparts to use physician services, although the differential went in the opposite direction with

Table 5.5   NHS Unadjusted Measures of Hospice Physician and Outpatient Utilization and Costs for Non-Medicare and Medicare Patients

	Hospital Based (N = 523)	Home Care (N = 808)
OUTPATIENT SERVICES		
Percent of Patients Using Outpatient Services		
Medicare	14	24
Non-Medicare	23	30
Outpatient Cost per Hospice Day		
Medicare	$0.55	$1.80
Non-Medicare	$2.35	$2.11
PHYSICIAN SERVICES		
Percent of Patients Using Physicians' Services		
Medicare	74	73
Non-Medicare	83	69
Physician Cost per Hospice Day		
Medicare	$7.95	$8.61
Non-Medicare	$8.98	$6.44

respect to outpatient services. The net result in terms of physician and outpatient service costs reveals fairly similar costs per day across all groups—about $8.50 to $11.50 per hospice day.

Out-of-Pocket Expenditures

The National Hospice Study gathered information about patients' and their families' out-of-pocket expenditures while receiving hospice care. These data were obtained from records maintained by patients' family members while the patient was alive and were assembled approximately four months after the death of the patient as a part of a scheduled bereavement interview. One reason for assembling service-utilization and charge data well after the patient died was to allow time for the family members to reconcile health-care bills with their insurance companies. Many families have multiple insurance policies and separate coverage for a portion of even Medicare copayments. This complexity makes it difficult to accurately determine the amount of out-of-pocket expenses actually paid by the patient and family.

In assembling our data, we asked the patients' family members the proportion of a particular bill that they did not expect their insurance company to cover. We also asked specifically about expenditures for items such as drugs, supplies, and equipment that the patients or family members had to pay for out of pocket. Both types of expenditures were discussed at each follow-up interview contact and were then reviewed and "reconciled" at the bereavement interview.

Based upon the manner in which the data were collected, two separate measures of out-of-pocket expenditures were created: expenses for drugs, supplies, and equipment; and general out-of-pocket expenditures associated with medical services such as hospital care, nursing home care, home nursing, and physician and outpatient and other therapies delivered either at home or in an inpatient setting. It is possible to add the two types of out-of-pocket charges. However, out-of-pocket charges cannot be added to charges for services such as physician visits since the same visit charge has a "covered" and an "uncovered" component. In our prior discussion of physician services, the charges to which we were referring reflected the total visit charge. Consequently, when calculating total costs or charges, only expenditures for drugs, supplies, and equipment are added to inpatient, physician, and home-care service unit charges.

Table 5.6 reveals that home-care hospice patients were more likely to report having had out-of-pocket expenses for drugs, supplies, and equipment than was the case for hospital-based hospice patients. Non-Medicare patients in hospital-based hospices had somewhat higher expenses than did their Medicare counterparts, but no such payor source differential appears to have existed among home-care patients. It is clear, however, that among home-care and hospital-

Table 5.6   NHS Unadjusted Measures of Hospice Out-of-pocket
Expenditures for Drugs, Supplies, and Equipment (DSE) and
Total Expenditure for Non-Medicare and Medicare Patients

	Hospital Based (N = 523)	Home Care (N = 808)
DRUGS, SUPPLIES, AND EQUIPMENT		
Percent of Patients with Expenditure		
Medicare	33	73
Non-Medicare	44	72
Expenditures per Hospice Day		
Medicare	$0.82	$1.63
Non-Medicare	$1.34	$2.12
TOTAL OUT-OF-POCKET EXPENDITURE		
Percent of Patients with Expenditure		
Medicare	44	45
Non-Medicare	51	36
Expenditure per Hospice Day		
Medicare	$13.80	$6.05
Non-Medicare	$18.81	$5.17

based hospice patients who did have expenses, non-Medicare patients paid
more per hospice day than did Medicare patients. It is likely that the availability
of better insurance coverage among Medicare patients, particularly those in the
demonstration, resulted in lower out-of-pocket expenditures for drugs, supplies, and equipment. Indeed, under the demonstration, a special benefit of
outpatient drug coverage was available, which presumably also reduced the
relative costs of drugs to patients while at home.

The largest differential in drugs, supplies, and equipment expenditures can
be seen between home- and hospital-based hospices. Since these costs are
included as a part of inpatient hospital bills, this difference is probably related
to the greater likelihood of inpatient utilization rather than a difference in the
prevalence of receiving these types of services. It is interesting to note that out-
of-pocket expenditures are higher among non-Medicare patients, even among
hospital-based hospice patients, when they are at home and have to pay for
these services.

Out-of-pocket expenditures associated with payment of medical services are
about equally likely among home- and hospital-based Medicare hospice patients. However, among non-Medicare patients, home-care hospice patients are
less likely to have such expenses than are hospital-based hospice patients. This
finding may appear anomalous until we recognize that copayment of inpatient
and physician bills may represent the highest component of out-of-pocket
expenditures. As we have already seen, both types of services were more likely
to have been provided to hospital-based hospice patients. Indeed, this in-

terpretation is borne out by examining the differences in the expenditures per hospice day for Medicare and non-Medicare patients served in hospital-based and home-care hospices. While non-Medicare home-care hospice patients have expenditures that are almost $1 less per hospice day than do Medicare patients, among hospital-based hospice patients, non-Medicare patients' expenditures are $5 per day higher than those of Medicare patients. This differential appears to be attributable to payor source, which is reasonable since non-Medicare patients may have had higher copayments or less comprehensive insurance coverage than exists for Medicare patients, particularly those served in demonstration sites.

Examining the Effect of Demonstration Status on Cost and Services

The relative influence of Medicare status versus whether the patient received the benefits of the hospice demonstration project cannot be precisely determined. As we saw in chapter 2, demonstration hospices differed from nondemonstration hospices in several important ways that might have affected their costs and pattern of service delivery, not the least of which is that demonstration hospices were, for the most part, larger than nondemonstration hospices. Additionally, it is difficult to separate the effect of hospice type from demonstration status for the reasons cited in chapter 2. To further complicate matters, estimates for non-Medicare patients in demonstration hospices for each type of hospice are unstable in view of the relatively small number of nondemonstration hospice patients (under 300).

Despite these complications, this section briefly examines the various effects associated with demonstration status, taking into consideration both the differences attributable to hospice type and Medicare status. We focus upon the differentials associated with inpatient and home-care service use as well as the amount of out-of-pocket expenditures.

Tables 5.7 and 5.8 present the percent of users and costs per hospice day for inpatient and home care, broken down by hospice type and demonstration status. Payor source is also identified. Since the majority of patients in both

Table 5.7 Two Measures of Inpatient Service Utilization by Hospice Type, Demonstration Status, and Payor Source

	Demonstration		Nondemonstration	
	% Users	$/Hospice Day	% Users	$/Hospice Day
Hospital Based				
Total	82	90	89	147
Non-Medicare	83	82	87	129
Home Care				
Total	45	41	52	44
Non-Medicare	56	38	52	47

Table 5.8   Two Measures of Home-Care Use by Hospice Type, Demonstration Status, and Payor Source

	Demonstration		Nondemonstration	
	% Users	$/Hospice Day	% Users	$/Hospice Day
Hospital Based				
Total	67	50	54	32
Non-Medicare	63	35	63	35
Home Care				
Total	100	57	97	33
Non-Medicare	100	44	95	40

demonstration and nondemonstration settings were Medicare beneficiaries, the important aspect of the payor source breakdown is to enable comparisons across demonstration and nondemonstration hospices for non-Medicare as well as all patients.

The data indicate that demonstration and nondemonstration hospices of the same type make comparable use of inpatient services. This trend holds true whether or not non-Medicare patients are served. Additionally, the measures of costs per hospice day also exhibit substantial uniformity across demonstration status and payor source.

A more interesting pattern of findings emerges with respect to home-care services. Although the proportion of patients receiving any service appears fairly similar for all groups, in demonstration settings, non-Medicare patients receive a less intensive level of home-care services as measured by the cost per hospice. Additionally, demonstration patients received a more intensive home-care intervention. One of the principal reasons for the more intensive intervention is that demonstration hospice patients received longer visits, making them, on average, more costly than home services received by nondemonstration hospice patients. Among non-Medicare patients, no such demonstration effect appears to have been operating.

Earlier, in examining out-of-pocket expenditures, we observed costs to be higher among hospital-based hospice patients, particularly among non-Medicare patients. Upon closer examination, and taking into consideration demonstration status, we found that this difference was largely due to the very high out-of-pocket expenditures reported by nondemonstration hospital-based hospice patients, both Medicare and non-Medicare. Comparing demonstration hospital-based and home-care hospice patients' out-of-pocket expenses reveals that their costs per day were between $6 and $8 regardless of payor source. Among nondemonstration hospital-based hospice patients, the reported daily costs exceeded $40, while for home-care hospice patients, they were only around $10. It is not clear exactly why payor source made less of a difference in determining out-of-pocket expenditures than did demonstration status. However, it would appear that under the demonstration, patients' use of inpatient and home services with no copayment required resulted in relatively low out-of-pocket costs for a period of very intensive medical-care utilization.

Cost Savings in the Last Nine Weeks of Life

Regardless of the benefits associated with improved quality of life for patients or families, hospice care is a less expensive mode of treatment if comparable patients cost less in hospice than in conventional care. Findings reported in chapter 4 show that hospice care yielded savings for demonstration patients after adjusting for patient mix differences, particularly in the last one or two months of life. However, the size of these savings was shown to depend heavily on patients' length of stay in the hospice and on levels of utilization prior to hospice intake. For very long stays, particularly among hospital-based hospice patients, the cumulative savings of hospice care became negative; that is, hospice care costs more than conventional care for patients with stays greater than two months who received care in hospital-based hospices.

In this section, we estimate hospice savings in total service costs over the last nine weeks of life. This completes the savings analysis begun in chapter 4 by describing detailed utilization patterns within the last months of life. Although analyses of these data have certain limitations associated with small sample sizes and relatively restricted data on prior service use, it was encouraging to find that these analyses supported the findings that hospices are cost effective relative to conventional care, as reported in chapter 4. Findings are presented in two formats. First, the pattern of cost and utilization differences between the two modes of hospice and conventional care are presented, and second, estimates of total cost savings per study day during approximately the last fifty days of life are presented.

Costs and Utilization in the Last Sixty-three Days of Life

Figure 5.1 shows patterns of inpatient and home-care utilization in the last sixty-three days of life. Levels of inpatient use, measured in days, were similar in hospital-based hospice and conventional-care settings during all periods, though numerical values for hospital-based hospice patients were lower in each case.

The inpatient cost differential between these groups (see table 5.9) was determined more by higher ancillary costs per inpatient day in conventional-care hospitals than by frequency and lengths of inpatient stay. Figure 5.1 also shows that home-care patients used considerably fewer inpatient days in each period than either hospital-based hospice or conventional-care patients. Thus, even though average inpatient utilization increased nearly threefold from the

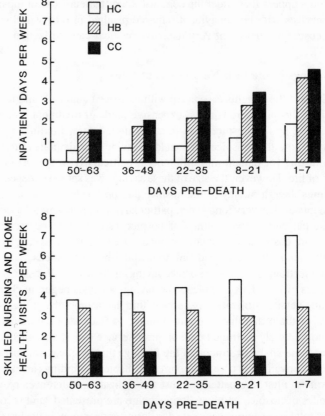

Figure 5.1   Patterns of Utilization of Home-Care and Hospital-Based Hospices of Follow-up Sample Members as Death Approached by Treatment Setting

period fifty to sixty-three days before death to the last week of life in all three settings, inpatient utilization of home-care patients remained about one-half the level shown in the other two settings.

Use of home-care services was consistently lower in conventional care than in either hospice setting; moreover, this rate showed no tendency to increase or decrease as death approached. In contrast, use of both skilled nursing and home health services increased as home-care hospice patients approached death. Hospital-based hospice patients apparently added home care, particularly skilled nursing, onto increasing levels of inpatient utilization. Utilization rates were nearly the same for both skilled nursing and home health in both hospice settings sixty-three days before death. Both conventional-care and hospital-based hospice patients increased their use of inpatient care. However, home-care hospice patients' use of home care increased to the point that in the last week of life they were receiving more than one visit per day.

Table 5.9   NHS Unadjusted Costs per Week in the Last Sixty-Three Days of Life in Home Care, Hospital-Based Hospice, and Conventional Care

	Setting		
Days before Death	Home-Care Hospice (N = 768)	Hospital-Based Hospice (N = 563)	Conventional Care (N = 290)
7 to 0	$1,042	$1,154	$1,290
21 to 8	665	859	808
35 to 22	543	748	527
49 to 36	516	629	296
63 to 50	460	581	176

The fact that the hospital-based hospice did not end up costing more than conventional care was due to differences in costs incurred in the last week of life. As can be seen in table 5.9, conventional-care costs rose dramatically, from a weekly average of $808 just prior to the last week to $1,290 in the last week, well above the $1,158 incurred by hospital-based hospice patients. Savings in home-care sites accrued through twenty-one days before death. In the period twenty-two to thirty-five days before death, home care was slightly more expensive than conventional care ($554, compared to $527). The excess costs of hospice care widened in earlier periods for both hospice types.

Total Cost Saving

Table 5.10 compares conventional-care costs per study day with those of home-care and hospital-based hospice patients, adjusting for the mix of patients in the group and their prior service use. These data clearly show that hospital-based hospices resembled conventional care in total cost, even though shares of inpatient and home-care costs differed between the settings. Both conventional-care and hospital-based hospice patients averaged over 40 percent higher costs per study day than patients in home care. However, inpatient costs per day were higher in conventional care ($135, compared to $99 for hospital-based hospice patients). Home-care costs incurred by hospital-based hospice patients were considerably higher than conventional home-care costs ($46, compared to $6).

Thus, patients in hospital-based hospice settings received the levels of home-care use associated with hospice care while maintaining a fairly high level of inpatient utilization. Hospital-based hospice programs added home care onto inpatient care, with the result that they showed no saving, on average, over conventional care.

Physician costs per day in both hospice settings were about one-half the level in conventional care. Hospice outpatient costs were lower as well, although patients in home-care hospices incurred higher expenses associated with clinic visits than did hospital-based hospice patients. Both hospital-based hospice and

Table 5.10   NHS Adjusted Estimates of Total Costs and Components per Study Day for Home-Care, Hospital-Based Hospice, and Conventional-Care Patients

	Setting		
Cost Category	Home-Care Hospice (N = 768)	Hospital-Based Hospice (N = 563)	Conventional Care (N = 290)
Inpatient costs per study day	$ 46 (8.8)	$ 99 (9.6)	$135 (11.6)
Home-care costs per study day	54 (4.5)	46 (4.9)	6 (1.1)
Physician costs per study day	9 (1.7)	8 (1.9)	18 (1.6)
Outpatient costs per study day	1.81 (0.69)	1.18 (0.75)	3.03 (0.84)
Drugs, supplies, and equipment costs per study day	1.82 (0.51)	0.73 (0.56)	0.11 (0.60)
Total costs per study day	101 (9.1)	146 (10.0)	149 (11.7)

Note: Numbers in parentheses are standard errors.

conventional-care patients spent less per day on drugs and supplies than home-care patients. This finding does not mean that home-care patients used more drugs and supplies than other patients; it means only that home-care patients spent more out of pocket on these items than other patients who received drugs and supplies while hospitalized.

These findings generally confirm estimates based on Medicare bills reported in chapter 4, which showed that over the long run hospital-based hospices do not yield cost savings but home-care hospices generally do. In spite of low "intensity" of inpatient ancillary use in hospital-based hospices, the combination of high inpatient utilization and high levels of home-care use throughout the sixty-three days before death make care in this setting more expensive than conventional care up to the last week of life. Home care proved to be less costly over a longer period.

Conclusion

One might argue, using these results, that the demonstration encouraged home care and discouraged inpatient care. The argument for a "home-care effect" is particularly strong. The average number of visits per week was higher in home-care and hospital-based demonstration hospices than in conventional care or in nondemonstration hospices. However, we cannot show that a demonstration effect actually occurred because we cannot screen out or control for characteristics of hospices that might predispose certain facilities to higher-than-average use of home or inpatient care. The sample of hospice sites in the NHS was too small to reliably estimate facility effects on utilization, and the relatively small number of nondemonstration hospice patients, when broken down by hospice type and payor source, made reliable estimation of the payor-source effect difficult.

Non-Medicare patients used less inpatient and home care than the average hospice patient. If the coverage that non-Medicare payors extend to hospice care remains the same in the next few years, then non-Medicare patients should continue to use fewer services than Medicare patients. However, if non-Medicare payors liberalize coverage, extending home-care benefits in particular, costs among non-Medicare patients can be expected to rise relative to the average.

The response of non-Medicare payors may be important to the long run viability of TEFRA's hospice benefit. Hospital-based hospices, faced with overhead costs that make participation in the Medicare program uneconomical, might seek certification more readily if some of the expected losses incurred serving Medicare patients could be recouped through higher charges to non-Medicare payors. An alternative solution that should prove more attractive to providers and insurers would be an agreement to accept some form of prospective rate setting that preserves equity in pricing across payors.

Home-care hospices were shown to be less costly than hospital-based hospices, regardless of demonstration status or payor category. The fact that many hospital-based hospice patients were essentially institution-bound throughout their stays contributed to this outcome. However, even those patients in hospital-based hospice facilities who used both inpatient and home care were more likely to be institutionalized, and to use more inpatient care, than the average home-care patient. The case for hospital-based hospice care, as it is portrayed in these pages, must rest on a determination that higher-cost institutional care may be appropriate for medically needy patients, rather than on the argument that hospice care is less expensive than conventional care. This argument should logically be predicated on the assumption that hospital-based hospices serve a different type of patient or that they can more effectively deliver some aspect of the hospice model of care. Whether or not this is true is examined in the next chapters.

6

The Medical and Social Service Interventions of Hospice and Nonhospice Patients

VINCENT MOR, DAVID S. GREER, AND RICHARD GOLDBERG

As we have seen, the hospice model of care takes a variety of forms. Some hospices are hospital based; others are freestanding organizations in the community. The range of services offered also varies to some extent from hospice to hospice. Nevertheless, all are guided by the same philosophy. All emphasize palliation as a principal therapeutic goal, and all attempt to provide support for patients and their families in the home. We have already seen substantial differences in the level of home services used by hospice and nonhospice cancer patients in the last months of life. The provision of counseling, self-care training, and other social service activities is also consistent with the hospice philosophy.

The hospice movement has grown rapidly over the past ten years; its message has been directed not only at care providers who have adopted the hospice system of care but also at the larger medical-care system (Saunders 1978; Stoddard 1978). The proliferation of hospices is an outgrowth of the movement but not its only manifestation. An original goal of the movement was to change the approach to caring for the terminally ill in the larger health-care system (Lunt and Hillier 1981). Indeed, the medical and nursing literature has begun to reflect many of the same values and approaches to pain and symptom control that were initially promulgated by the hospice movement (Shimm et al. 1979; Twycross 1977). Consequently, conventional care may already have begun to approximate aspects of hospice care.

The conceptual framework guiding our evaluation posited that the hospice movement would achieve its goal of improving patient outcomes by altering the traditional pattern of care. We recognized that changing the pattern of care would not be easy, particularly in settings where the hospice did not control all aspects of the care prescribed for the patient. We also suspected that changes in philosophy and pattern of care were also occurring in the conventional-care system. To determine whether the care provided hospice and nonhospice patients was different, we compared patients' receipt of a variety of medical and social services during the last weeks of life.

This chapter explores similarities and differences in the nature and pattern of care received by hospice and nonhospice patients. Observed differences may reflect either variations in the treatment philosophy associated with the type of setting (HC, HB, CC) *or* differences in the choices made by patients and their families. We have already seen that patients who elected HC hospices had a predisposition to use home care prior to hospice entry, while HB patients had a predisposition to have lower inpatient ancillary costs per day. These preexisting differences can be presumed to carry over into the pattern of terminal care provided. Despite these differences, however, the importance of the setting itself should not be underestimated. Underlying the option to choose hospice care or conventional care is the expectation that the type and level of treatment will meet the particular preferences of patient and family. Should it prove that treatment patterns do *not* vary significantly across settings, then the choice of setting would provide only the illusion of control. Hospice care, for example, would not represent a clear alternative if aggressive procedures (see below) were carried out as frequently as in conventional care, despite the patient and family expectations. The services received by hospice and nonhospice patients can be regarded as the outcome of interactions between patient-family choice and predisposition and the prevailing philosophy and practice of the setting.

This chapter, then, examines the key question of whether patients of comparable clinical status receive similar or differential medical and social service interventions in the three treatment settings.

The comparisons focus on the clinical choices made during the terminal phase of illness. Should aggressive treatment be continued, or should the emphasis shift to palliation and supportive social services? In practice, these decisions are complex and individual. One cannot assume that all the factors involved are given equal consideration. Furthermore, it is possible that some decisions are "made" by the care provider's philosophy without explicit conscious deliberation.

As described in chapter 3, the NHS collected data about a broad array of services. We chose to classify these services as falling into one of four groups: aggressive therapies, diagnostic testing, supportive-palliative services, and social services. We recognize that the line between aggressive and palliative services with an end-stage cancer patient may not always be clear. Radiation therapy, surgery, and even chemotherapy may be introduced for palliation. Nevertheless, we felt that it was appropriate to infer that differences in service receipt across settings, adjusting for clinical differences in the types of patients served, did reflect differences in treatment philosophy.

Data used for comparing services received included the interviews with PCPs, inpatient records, medication reviews with PCPs, records of patients' prescriptions and how they were consumed, and adjusted Medicare billing data (to characterize ancillary use during inpatient stays). For the most part, analyses compared the proportions of patients receiving a given service at some point approximately one to five weeks prior to death. As described in chapter 3, we adjusted the comparisons whenever appropriate to take into consideration certain known differences between the hospice and conventional-care patients. In some instances, however, the more appropriate method of comparison was to focus on a subgroup of medically homogeneous patients and examine observed differences in the mode of response of the treatment setting to the onset of a particular symptom. These clinical profiles were developed by oncologists and radiation oncology specialists with many years of clinical and research experience in these areas. In the sections that follow, we differentiate the samples upon which the results were based in order to provide a context for the reader.

Aggressive Therapies

One of the principal features that presumably differentiates the hospice philosophy from prevailing medical practice is the definition of when curative therapy should cease (Saunders 1978). This may be in part a reflection of how ready the medical-care provider is to interpret symptoms and response to therapy as indicative of poor prognosis. Attention to the signs of decline and a belief that ministrations outside the realm of curative therapy are also valuable may be the important determinant of hospice-versus-nonhospice medical practice (Cassileth 1979).

Each patient's PCP was asked whether or not the physician seemed to favor aggressive antitumor therapy. Over 35 percent of CC patients' physicians were characterized as "aggressive" in treating the patient, while this was true for only 14 percent and 22 percent of the HB and HC groups, respectively. At this juncture in the care of the patients (between forty and fifty days prior to death), the perspective of the physician who is legally responsible for prescribing all care may be crucial. While physicians of hospice patients were significantly less likely to be seen as aggressive than were those of CC patients, we should recall that the personal physician is rarely a "hospice physician" or the hospice medical director. Most hospice patients continue their ongoing relationship with the physician who had been treating them prior to the choice of hospice care. Therefore, it is not surprising that some hospice patients' physicians are characterized as aggressive. What is encouraging from the perspective of the evaluation was that only one-third of CC patients' physicians were so characterized. Since none of these physicians was affiliated with a hospice, it may be that aggressiveness diminishes naturally as the patient deteriorates. Indeed,

Table 6.1   Percentage of Patients Receiving Aggressive Interventions in the Last Measure prior to Death

	Home Care	Hospital Based	Conventional Care	Probability of Chi-Square
Aggressive Interventions (any one of the services listed below)	13.9	13.1	37.7	<0.001
Surgery	0.6	1.9	6.8	<0.001
Chemo or hormone therapy	7.2	5.4	24.2	<0.001
Radiation therapy	3.8	5.6	13.5	<0.001
Thoracocentesis	4.3	2.9	6.8	0.18

how aggressive the physician is perceived to be is an important corollary of whether aggressive care is provided.

Table 6.1 presents the percentage of sample members who received various intensive interventions at the last measure before death. As can be seen, CC patients were significantly more likely to receive any of the medical interventions characterized as intensive. The principal service contributing to the composite measure was chemotherapy. It was in this area that the largest percentage difference between hospice care and conventional care was found, although receipt of all services but thoracocentesis (a procedure employed for draining air or fluid from the space around the lungs) was significantly more likely among conventional-care than hospice patients.

Even before patients entered a hospice, they were less likely to have received intensive services than were conventional-care patients (63.4 percent CC versus 34.9 percent and 42.8 percent for HB and HC patients, respectively). If hospice and conventional-care patients started out so differently, then it is difficult to accept the position that lower use of aggressive care in the last weeks of life is attributable to hospice care rather than to a predisposition to avoid such services. To address this issue, we compared the percentage of patients who started the study receiving aggressive care and were still using it in the last weeks before death across hospice and conventional-care groups. While 40.7 percent of conventional-care patients who initially were receiving aggressive care were still receiving it during the last weeks before death, this was true for only 23.9 percent and 17.1 percent of home-care and hospital-based patients respectively ($p < .005$). These data, in conjunction with the initial and final measure comparisons, suggest that as death approached all three groups were less likely to receive intensive interventions; however, hospice patients were still much less likely to receive such services than were conventional-care patients. As will be seen later in this chapter, decreases in use of aggressive care were not paralleled by increases in respiratory or other definitely supportive therapies as patients approached death. Nonetheless, we do assume that palliative activities of some form increased.

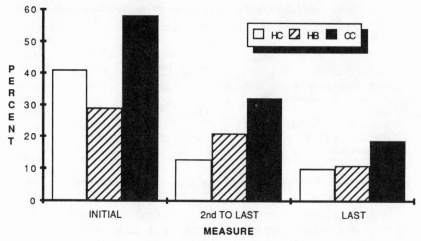

Figure 6.1   Estimated Receipt of Aggressive Services by Time prior to Death

Statistical models were developed to estimate the likelihood of receiving aggressive services in each setting for three different time periods: last, second to last, and around study entry. The estimated probability was developed by applying the characteristics of the average demonstration hospice patient to each model. This estimate was akin to asking how a hospice patient with a given set of characteristics would respond in one of the three settings had he or she been served there.

As can be seen in figure 6.1, although at the last measurement period conventional-care patients are still more likely to have received aggressive care, the observed difference is not statistically significant after adjusting for patient characteristics. The trend, however, suggests that clinically similar patients would be treated differently in a hospice than they would be in conventional care. The figure also reveals that home-care patients' receipt of aggressive care drops most rapidly from the initial to the last measure.

Examining the relationship between patient characteristics and the probability of receiving aggressive services revealed that older patients were less likely to receive aggressive care than were younger patients. Furthermore, if the patient's PCP were younger, then the patient was more likely to get aggressive care. Additionally, patients with breast cancer were more likely to be treated aggressively, which, given the beliefs and data about breast cancer's being curable, is understandable. Finally, patients whose PCPs characterized the physician as aggressive were much more likely to actually receive aggressive services ($p < .01$). In summary, then, younger patients, those with younger PCPs, those with breast cancer, or those with aggressive physicians were more likely to receive aggressive treatments, particularly in nonhospice settings.

Inpatient Ancillary Services

Another approach to examining treatment patterns that can be used is related to the relative "intensity" of the ancillary services patients receive while in an inpatient setting. When patients are hospitalized or placed into an inpatient setting, the cost of the care they receive can be defined in terms of routine inpatient room-and-board services, including regular nursing care. Another component of the nonphysician costs are those associated with "ancillary" services, ranging from the cost of the operating room to the cost of inhalation therapy or pharmaceuticals and diagnostic tests. In relation to the cost analyses described earlier, we standardized all inpatient bills of all Medicare patients in our study served in either hospice or nonhospice settings. The standardization consisted of adjusting for the relative costliness of each hospital serving a study patient nationally and then adjusting for the propensity of each hospital to provide a high or low level of ancillary services. The resulting measure of ancillary costs per inpatient day reflects the relative intensity of the pattern of services provided a study patient during a hospitalization.

Data provided by the family members can be validated by comparing the level of ancillary costs per inpatient day during the last month of life across the three treatment settings. This approach does not account for the large proportion of hospice home-care patients who did not enter an inpatient setting at all during their care under a hospice. We examined all hospice patients' service use in hospice for at least thirty days, meaning that any inpatient admission during this period was associated with their care under the supervision of the hospice, and compared the intensity of services provided them to that of nonhospice patients as reflected in the ancillary costs per inpatient day. The HC patients had ancillary costs per day of $98 versus $67 for HB patients and $184 for CC patients. The higher intensity of intervention in conventional care corroborates the findings presented earlier. That HB patients had higher costs than HC patients may be a reflection of the fact that HB hospices had less control over the course of the care their patients received once admitted to an inpatient setting.

The Use of Diagnostic Tests

Another less well defined measure of the invasiveness of medical technology for the terminally ill is exposure to the myriad diagnostic tests that the medical system regularly dispenses, particularly to patients in an inpatient setting. This section compares the probability of receiving diagnostic tests among hospice and nonhospice patients. Diagnostic tests vary considerably both in terms of their invasiveness and their utility for terminal patients. In most instances, admission to a hospital requires a battery of tests as a matter of policy. Depending upon the type of setting, many other tests are routinely ordered and undertaken on a daily basis as physicians investigate fluctuations in patients' vital signs and symptoms reported by the patient, the patient's family, or the nursing staff. Comparing the prevalence of various diagnostic tests across hospice and non-hospice patients provides a further indication of the philosophy of the systems offering care to the terminally ill patient.

Data for these comparisons were obtained exclusively from the patients' primary care persons. We were able to ascertain information reliably only about blood tests and X rays or other scans. These two tests are easily identified by nonmedical persons. No effort was made to determine the frequency of such tests over a given time frame, since blood can be drawn serially for multiple types of tests at various points in the day or all at once. Since such tests can be administered on an outpatient basis and in the hospital, we relied upon the PCP to provide the information regardless of where the patient was.

The percentage of patients who received one or the other of the two diagnostic tests at the time of our last interview was 72 percent for CC patients as opposed to 36 percent and 38 percent for HB and HC patients, respectively. At study entry, CC patients were almost unanimous in reporting receipt of diagnostic tests in the prior two weeks. At the same point in time, some three-quarters of HB and HC patients also received diagnostic tests. The proportion of patients receiving tests dropped in all groups as deterioration progressed. Nonetheless, the rate of decline of diagnostic test use was considerably sharper among hospice than nonhospice patients. Among patients who reported receiving one or the other of the two tests around the time of study entry, 55 percent and 71 percent of the HC and HB hospice patients, respectively, no longer received such tests in the last weeks of life. For CC patients, only 31 percent receiving tests at the outset were no longer receiving them in the last weeks before death. This difference is highly significant statistically ($p > .001$), suggesting that the nonhospice patient setting continued to engage in more intrusive interventions, perhaps only for the purpose of adhering to established procedures.

Statistical models were developed to estimate the likelihood of the average hospice patient's receiving diagnostic tests at the last and second-to-last measures prior to death. A similar model was developed to estimate diagnostic test use prior to the initial interview contact. The results of statistically adjusted estimates of diagnostic test use are summarized in figure 6.2. As can be seen, the average hospice patient was significantly less likely to receive diagnostic tests at any of the three measures if served in either of the hospice settings than if served in a CC setting. The estimated probability of receiving diagnostic tests was virtually identical in HB and HC hospices.

We examined the statistical model developed to test differences in the use of diagnostic tests in order to describe the factors that influenced their use. Younger patients were significantly more likely to have received a diagnostic test than were older patients, regardless of the type of setting. Once again, whether or not the physician was viewed as aggressive was strongly related to receipt of

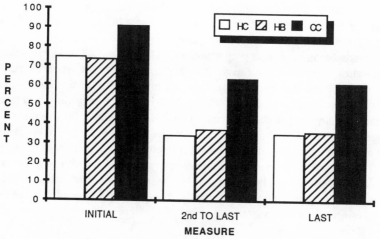

Figure 6.2   Estimated Receipt of Diagnostic Tests by Time prior to Death

diagnostic tests. Interestingly, neither cancer type nor area of metastasis was consistently related to use of diagnostic tests.

The Use of Supportive and Palliative Services

A hallmark of the hospice philosophy is the focus upon supportive medical therapies that are largely palliative in nature. This chapter separately assesses the uses of medical supportive therapies and nonmedical interventions. The range of medical therapies that can be considered supportive or palliative is considerable and can include certain services that we have included as aggressive in the discussions above. In selecting the types of services that we felt could be reasonably defined as palliative, we restricted ourselves to those areas in which we felt we could gather valid data. We developed a mixed strategy, collecting information about respiratory therapy and oxygen use, both decidedly supportive medical interventions, from PCPs of all sample members and selected data about medication use from a smaller subsample of patients. We also developed a series of clinically relevant conditions in which the prevalence of selected interventions that might be clinically indicated were compared by treatment setting. These analyses relied on specified subsets of the larger follow-up sample used in all comparisons presented above.

This section first presents general comparisons of the use of supportive respiratory services such as respiratory therapy and oxygen. Respiratory therapy is generally performed by skilled technicians in an inpatient setting, while oxygen can also be used at home. Both measures of each individual service as well as a combined indicator of receiving either respiratory therapy or oxygen are presented. This general comparison is followed by the results of selected clinical comparisons and then analyses of the rate of medication use of analgesics, antiemetics, and psychotropics.

At study entry, similar proportions of HC, HB, and CC patients reported receiving either oxygen or respiratory therapy (29 percent versus 27 percent versus 29 percent, respectively). The percentage of CC recipients increased between initial and last contact, while in both hospice settings the percentage of users remained around 30 percent. Of all CC patients who did not report receiving respiratory support at the initial measure, 27 percent received it at the final measure; this was true for only 11.3 percent and 19.5 percent of HC and HB patients. This difference was significant ($p = .02$). Oxygen administration was more common in all settings than was respiratory therapy. Indeed, most of those receiving respiratory therapy also received oxygen; respiratory therapy was rarely reported alone.

Respiratory Support

Table 6.2 presents data describing oxygen and respiratory therapy receipt by treatment setting as reported at the last measure prior to the patient's death. For each individual measure, as well as for the composite measure, CC patients were more likely to receive these services than were hospice patients, without adjusting for differences in the characteristics of the patients served in the three groups. Findings suggest that CC settings are more likely to respond with respiratory support to newly developing symptoms, whereas hospice settings may rely upon other approaches.

No statistical differences were found across the groups when the response of the average demonstration hospice patient was estimated by the equations developed by the NHS (see figure 6.3). The CC patients were somewhat more likely to receive either form of therapy at the last measure before death. This pattern was reversed, however, for the next-to-last measure, although again the estimates were not significantly different across treatment settings. These adjusted findings suggest that when hospice patients with comparable demographic, social support, and medical factors are seen in a conventional-care

Table 6.2   Percentage of Patients Receiving Respiratory Support in the Last Measure prior to Death

	Home Care	Hospital Based	Conventional Care	Probability of Chi-Square
Respiratory support intervention (any one of the services listed below)	32.2	27.2	44.0	<.001
Oxygen administration	30.0	26.1	42.8	<.001
Respiratory therapy	7.7	5.4	15.3	.003

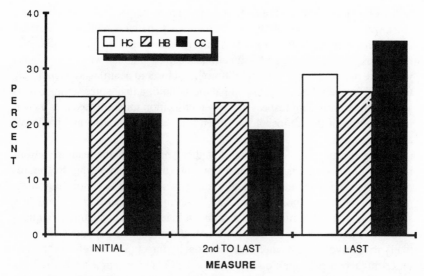

Figure 6.3   Estimated Receipt of Respiratory Support by Time prior to Death

setting, their treatment is similar to what they would have received in either type of hospice setting.

In an effort to understand what types of patients received respiratory support, we examined the equations used to statistically adjust the comparisons of patients served in the three different settings. In contrast to the types of services previously mentioned, respiratory support was almost exclusively related to the type of cancer and the organs involved in the metastasis; lung cancer patients and those with metastases to the pleura were significantly more likely to receive respiratory support independent of age, treatment setting, and performance status level. Since lung disease and involvement are primary determinants of shortness of breath (dyspnea), their strong relationship to the provision of respiratory support was expected.

Based upon this finding, a clinical profile analysis plan was developed to determine the probability of using either oxygen or respiratory therapy among patients with specific disease and symptom attributes relevant to respiratory problems. Specifically, patients with primary lung disease or lung metastases who reported shortness of breath were compared in terms of receipt of either oxygen or respiratory therapy concurrent with the occasion of the symptom.

Statistical analyses of the 595 patients with lung disease and with shortness of breath revealed that 18 percent of CC patients received respiratory therapy *subsequent* to the occasion of experiencing shortness of breath, as opposed to 10 percent and 7 percent of the HB and HC hospice patients ($p > .05$). However, there were no significant differences among the three treatment settings in terms of receipt of oxygen therapy around the time patients reported shortness of breath (41 percent, 39 percent, and 46 percent, respectively, for HC, HB, and CC patients). Interestingly, we found that CC patients reporting shortness of breath when they were relatively independent were much *less* likely to receive oxygen than comparably functional hospice patients, while CC patients who were in poorer functional condition (i.e., closer to death) were *more* likely to receive oxygen than those of comparable condition in hospice settings. This specific difference with respect to oxygen utilization might be taken as a clear manifestation of the philosophical difference between curative and palliative approaches.

Taking the two sets of findings together presents an interesting view of resource allocation decisions in the hospice and nonhospice setting. Respiratory therapy—the more technologically intensive approach to controlling shortness of breath—was preferred in the CC setting. Oxygen therapy, which is simple enough to be administered at home, was used with comparable frequency in both CC and hospice settings. The fact that hospice patients were more likely to receive oxygen when still functionally intact (and therefore earlier in the terminal course of their disease) than were CC patients presumably reflects the greater use of home care services, since most hospice patients functioning at that level were still at home. In general, then, these clinical findings confirm the analyses presented above concerning the use of either respiratory therapy or oxygen when similar patients are compared across the three settings.

Palliative Radiation Therapy

In an earlier section, we included receipt of radiation therapy as one of a series of aggressive treatments terminal cancer patients can receive. However, under various clinical conditions, radiation therapy is used for the purpose of palliation—for example, to shrink tumors causing symptoms that reduce patients' quality of life. In an effort to determine whether hospice and nonhospice interventions were different with respect to the provision of palliative radiation therapy, our oncology consultants constructed two clinical profiles under which there is general consensus as to the purposes for providing radiation therapy.

First, a clinical profile was specified for which palliation is generally not a priority (that is, among terminal cancer patients with primary disease of, or metastases to, the brain). Patients meeting this criterion across the three sites were compared in terms of the probability of receiving radiation therapy, controlling for their functional status at the time. It was assumed that patients functioning poorly would be less likely to receive radiation therapy whether for palliative or curative purposes.

The second profile specified included patients with bone metastases who reported having bone pain. Since radiation therapy is a preferred mode of relief of bone pain, we assumed that there would be no difference in the proportion of hospice and nonhospice patients receiving radiation therapy under these conditions.

Analyses of the 311 patients with brain metastases revealed that a significantly higher proportion of nonhospice than hospice patients received radiation therapy ($p > .001$). This finding was obtained for both poor- and well-functioning patients. Among the 192 patients who were functioning poorly (nearly bedbound) around the time they received radiation therapy, 30 percent of nonhospice patients received radiation therapy, as opposed to only 7 percent of hospice patients, whether or not they were in an inpatient setting.

A different pattern was observed when patients with bone metastases were compared. Of the 314 patients with bone metastases who reported bone pain, there were no statistically significant differences in the proportions of those who received radiation therapy across the three groups. Although poorly functioning nonhospice patients were somewhat more likely to receive radiation than their hospice counterparts, this was not true of the better-functioning patients. In neither of these cases, however, was the difference statistically significant.

These two sets of findings taken together suggest that hospices were not refraining from providing radiation therapy as a palliative intervention in our study, particularly among more functional patients. However, hospices tended to refrain from this approach to palliation for either brain or bone metastases among the patients who were sicker and closer to death. The nonhospice patients were substantially more likely to be exposed to this relatively aggressive approach to palliation at a point when they were functionally impaired and well along on the path of terminal deterioration. As we will see throughout the rest of this chapter, hospice care appears to have taken a slightly different tack in dealing with intractable symptoms.

Analgesic Prescriptions and Utilization Patterns

Pain control is one of the central goals of the hospice movement and, indeed, represents one of the significant ostensible differences in the medical technology used to care for the terminally ill (Saunders 1978; Twycross 1977; Twycross and Lack 1984). The founders of the hospice movement maintained that through the correct calibration of analgesic medications, using a scheduled, preventive approach instead of a reactive approach to analgesic administration and prescription, all but the most intractable types of pain from terminal cancer could be ameliorated (Mount 1976). Consequently, in our study, we felt it was important to be able to document the pattern of analgesic prescription and utilization among hospice and nonhospice patients.

To this end, selected medication data were obtained for a subsample of 181 patients. All medications about which information was gathered were categorized into analgesic and nonanalgesic prescriptions. Detailed information about each relevant prescribed medication was noted during each interview with patients and their primary caretakers. Included was the exact medication, dose, prescribed frequency of consumption, and the number of units actually consumed in the last twenty-four hours. Interviewers checked medication charts if patients were in an inpatient setting and reviewed the actual bottles of pills with respondents if the patient was at home. A conversion algorithm was developed to equate the dosage of all analgesic medications based upon the concept of an oral morphine equivalent (Goldberg et al. 1986). This allowed us to sum across a wide array of narcotic and nonnarcotic analgesics and compare the actual level of medication consumed by patients in addition to comparing the percentage of patients receiving and consuming analgesics. Analyses were performed in reference to when patients died as well as for the full period of their participation in the study.

Over the course of the study, 34 percent of the 181 patients in the sample had a prescription for morphine, 20 percent had one for Dilaudid, and 12 percent had one for Percocet. Interestingly, Tylenol with codeine was prescribed for 16 percent of the patients, and 13 percent had a prescription for regular Tylenol. This latter figure is in addition to the many patients presumed to be taking some form of aspirin without a prescription.

Comparing hospice and nonhospice patients, we found that HB hospice patients were significantly more likely to have had an analgesic prescribed at the last measure before their death than was the case for either nonhospice or HC hospice patients ($p < .05$). Ninety-one percent of HB patients had an analgesic prescribed at the last measure versus 66 percent and 70 percent of the HC and nonhospice groups, respectively. A similar finding was observed with respect to patients actually taking the analgesic prescribed: 78 percent of HB versus 66 percent of HC and 57 percent of nonhospice patients ($p < .05$). While HB hospice patients were more likely to take analgesics, the average oral morphine equivalent level consumed per patient day was *not* significantly different across the three groups. On the other hand, nonhospice patients were more likely to have prescriptions that were for analgesics administered on an "as needed" basis and were less likely to have their analgesics prescribed orally than was the case for either type of hospice patient.

The observed differences, though small, suggest that nonhospice patients do not receive analgesics until their need for pain relief is relatively high. This is indicated by the fact that nonhospice patients who received analgesics received relatively high doses but, as a group, were less likely to receive any analgesics at all. Additionally, differences in the mode of administration of analgesics are consistent with the hospice philosophy of not prescribing "PRN" (on an as-needed basis) and of making analgesics available via the oral route whenever possible.

The Use of Other Medications

Several other types of medications are routinely used to palliate or alleviate the untoward symptoms of terminal cancer patients. Information was gathered about patients' receipt of selected phenothiazine and antihistamine antiemetics. Since nausea and vomiting are prevalent symptoms reported by as many as half of terminal cancer patients regardless of whether they are receiving chemotherapy, the rate of utilization of these medications should shed additional light on differences in the pattern of medical intervention hospice and nonhospice patients receive. We also gathered data on the use of selected psychotropic medications because their use may reflect providers' sensitivity to mood states patients experience. The use of antiemetics and psychotropic medications for hospice and nonhospice patients is summarized below. In all cases, findings refer to the 181 patients included in the medication sample.

Antiemetic use was not confined to patients who reported being nauseous. Thirty-two percent of patients with nausea had an antiemetic prescribed, and so did 19 percent of patients without nausea. There was no difference in the percentage of patients either receiving or taking antiemetics as a function of treatment setting (Reuben and Mor 1986). Indeed, most patients who had an antiemetic prescription took the prescribed medicine whether at home or in an inpatient setting. Elderly patients were significantly less likely to have an antiemetic prescribed, both among those with and without nausea. Perhaps the most important aspect of these analyses was our finding that less than one-third of patients with nausea had an antiemetic prescribed. This suggests that the physicians of terminal cancer patients should be more attuned to this symptom among their patients whether they are in a hospice or nonhospice setting.

Psychotropic medications were classified into several groups: antidepressants, barbiturates, benzodiazepines, and neuroleptics. This latter category was largely accounted for by antiemetic medications, and those drugs explicitly used as antiemetics were included only in the antiemetic analyses discussed above. Only 3 percent of patients consumed antidepressants, 7 percent used barbiturates, 1 percent consumed sedative-hypnotics, and 7 percent used neuroleptics that were not specifically used as antiemetics (Goldberg and Mor 1985). Given the low usage rates for each of these types of psychotropics, it is not surprising that we found no differences as a function of treatment setting. Hospice patients were no more likely to use psychotropics than were nonhospice patients. This lack of difference does not imply any normative standard; the hospice philosophy does not particularly advocate the use of psychotropics one way or the other. The low use of antidepressants does suggest, however, that psychiatric input is probably limited in the provision of medical care to terminally ill cancer patients. Whether this is appropriate would require a more detailed examination of mood state and psychiatric symptomatology than was possible in our study. It is to be hoped that future studies will be able to examine the relationship between terminal cancer and nonsomatic psychiatric symptoms.

Intravenous Care and Transfusions

In the final weeks of life, terminal cancer patients are frequently barraged with a broad array of therapies that are provided as a "last ditch" effort to cause the tumor to shrink and in so doing slightly extend life for the patient. These therapies frequently require some form of intravenous intervention, ranging from the administration of chemotherapies or infusions to simple hydration or blood transfusion in the last stages of deterioration. The hospice philosophy has traditionally eschewed "heroic" efforts that prolong the length but diminish the quality of life of patients (DuBois 1980). The classic portrait of the impersonal, conventional medical setting is a terminal bedside scene replete with gastrointestinal tubes, hydration lines, and, not infrequently, blood transfusion bags. In contrast, the ideal final scene in the hospice ideology is a homelike environment without the technological symbols of medical activity (Kohut and Kohut 1984).

Since the NHS was not able to systematically characterize these scenes qualitatively during the final days of life, we relied upon the data routinely collected from each patient's primary care person as to whether the patient had received some form of intravenous care since the last time she or he was contacted. Additionally, for patients in the medication sample, we also determined whether the patient had received a transfusion in the intervening period between interview contacts. These data were used to address the most delicate and potentially biased aspect of the comparison of the hospice and nonhospice interventions—use of intravenous care (I.V.) and transfusions in connection with clinically identified needs during the final six weeks of life.

In the case of intravenous care, two clinical profiles were specified in order to compare the responses of hospice and conventional care to patient symptoms. First, patients with liver metastases reporting anorexia were compared in terms of likelihood of receiving I.V. care. Second, patients with liver metastases who were hemorrhaging were compared to see what proportions had received I.V. care around the time they were hemorrhaging. Liver metastasis was chosen since such patients have an acknowledgedly poor prognosis, and yet, all other things being equal, will not have numerous complex and discomforting symptoms. In order to better understand the relationship of these comparisons to patients' proximity to death, we independently examined reasonably well functioning and very sick patients.

Figure 6.4 presents the proportion of patients with the two clinical conditions who received I.V. care concurrent with reporting the relevant symptom by treatment setting. As can be seen, nonhospice patients were significantly more likely to report I.V. use in both scenarios. Among low-functioning patients with anorexia, those in the nonhospice treatment group were over twice as likely to

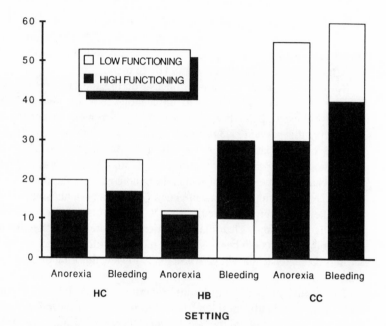

Figure 6.4   Receipt of Intravenous Care by Setting

have I.V. use as were HC or HB patients. As expected, I.V. use was more prevalent among low-functioning than among higher-functioning patients; however, almost all of that difference is attributable to the substantial difference in I.V. use among low- and high-functioning nonhospice patients.

Intravenous use did not define the content of the I.V. solution administered to the patients. Intravenous care could consist of simple glucose and water, blood, or chemotherapy. Unfortunately, it was not possible to obtain data at that level of detail. It should be noted, however, that 30 percent of the CC patients meeting the anorexia clinical condition received chemotherapy, whereas this was the case for only 15 percent of HB patients and 17 percent of HC patients. The net result is that nonhospice patients were more likely to have I.V. care for chemotherapy than for other purposes.

The proportion of low-functioning, hemorrhaging CC patients who reported I.V. use was substantially higher than that of both the HB and HC patient groups. While the number of cases in the well-functioning group was small, the overall comparison yielded a significant difference across treatment settings ($p < .001$). Consistent with the clinical picture of patients with liver metastases who were hemorrhaging, almost all had died by the subsequent follow-up period.

This comparison provides another indication of the difference in the orientation of care for terminal cancer patients, particularly in comparing CC and HB patients. Both groups of patients were likely to be spending their last days in an inpatient setting. In such settings, it is generally standard procedure to maintain some form of intravenous care, if only a glucose solution drip. Clearly, that pattern of care was not carried out in HB settings.

Results of analyses of transfusion use during the last six weeks of life parallel the findings pertaining to intravenous-care use (Wachtel and Mor 1985). Nonhospice patients were nearly five times as likely to receive a transfusion during this period (27.3 percent versus 7.6 percent and 4.2 percent for HC and HB hospice patients, respectively; $p < .001$). Interestingly, receipt of transfusion among the patients in the medication sample was not related to patient characteristics such as cancer type or demographic factors such as age or sex. This finding suggests that, in general, patients in nonhospice settings are more likely to receive interventions such as transfusion at a time when it is becoming increasingly clear that the patient is unlikely to survive the disease. While transfusion could be considered a mode of palliation, patients in hospice settings have physicians who are less likely to view this kind of intervention as palliative.

The results of our comparisons regarding use of I.V. and transfusion therapies, traditionally considered to be "life-giving" interventions, are particularly important in light of the fact that there were no differences in the survival rates of hospice and nonhospice patients. This finding was corroborated by a well-controlled experiment (Kane et al. 1984) of hospice-versus-conventional terminal care in a Veterans Administration hospital. This suggests that the added interventions did not extend life. Whether they were associated with any benefits or costs in terms of patients' well-being and quality of life is discussed in the following chapter.

Receipt of Social and Alternate Service Interventions

A hallmark of the hospice movement, particularly in the United States, is the attention given to the psychosocial needs of terminally ill patients as well as to their medical and nursing-care needs. Additionally, given the frequently complex interagency relationships that characterize hospices in America, the role of social service personnel is crucial in coordinating the plan of care and communicating the changing needs of the patient to all members of the team. This section presents information comparing the pattern of utilization of social services reported by hospice and nonhospice patients over the last weeks and months of life. As with most other types of services, data were obtained from patients' family members. Social services may be provided by a variety of different types of staff, including volunteers. Consequently, we chose to determine whether patients had various discrete functions and activities provided for them, regardless of who provided the service. The comparisons presented

Table 6.3 Percentage of Patients Receiving Social Service Intervention in the Last Measure prior to Death and for the Study Period

Last Weeks of Life	Home Care	Hospital Based	Conventional Care	Significance of Difference
Social service intervention (one of the services listed below)	60.1	63.5	51.2	.007
General counseling	34.6	34.0	26.6	.073
Legal/financial counseling	8.0	8.0	7.6	.972
Paperwork/assistance	29.3	35.1	20.8	<.001
Help getting services	28.1	32.0	23.5	.069
Self-care training	7.7	9.7	6.4	.315
Total Study Period				
Social service intervention (one of the services listed below)	77.3	77.3	67.8	.004
General counseling	48.4	50.2	38.6	.005
Legal/financial counseling	13.4	13.6	13.4	.995
Paperwork/assistance	43.3	44.3	30.7	<.001
Help getting services	45.9	50.0	35.3	<.001
Self-care training	17.7	20.1	16.1	.371

below rely upon these data to display the proportion of patients in each setting who received some form of social services.

Table 6.3 presents the percentage of patients reporting receipt of a composite social service measure as well as its components at the last measure prior to death and for the total study period. As can be seen, nonhospice patients were significantly less likely than hospice patients to receive social service interventions in the last weeks of life and during the total period. This difference, however, was not seen in all of the specific service areas. Less than 10 percent of all three groups reported having received financial or legal counseling in the last weeks before death. Similarly, these two activities were less prevalent in the total study period. The largest area of difference pertained to general counseling and the provision of assistance with paperwork. Given the complexities of terminal patients' insurance claims, medical bills, and the multitude of forms pertaining to service eligibility, assistance in this area may have particular instrumental value for patients and their families. Of interest was the comparatively high percentage of nonhospice patients who received help obtaining services at this late stage in their lives. Understandably, the provision of self-care training at this stage of the patient's life was relatively rare in all groups; however, the cumulative study period measure did indicate that HB and HC patients were likely to receive services in this area earlier than was the case for nonhospice patients.

Prior to study entry, HB and HC patients were significantly more likely to receive one of the social service intervention components (83.6 percent HC; 79.7 percent HB; 47.6 percent CC). The three components that showed the greatest difference were general counseling, assistance with paperwork, and help getting services. The other two components were not significantly different among the three groups for the period. The differences observed prior to study entry may logically have been related to the process of applying for and being admitted to the hospice program. Most participating hospices conduct initial assessment visits *before* the patient is formally admitted to the program. The assessment often consists of problem solving with patients and their families regarding areas of needed assistance and the choices facing them. If the patient is to be admitted, service arrangements are often initiated immediately. Consequently, there was sound reason to expect that the differences observed in social service receipt were a part of the hospice program and not a result of it.

Examining differences in the transition from receipt to nonreceipt of social services between the initial and final measures revealed that nonhospice patients who initially received social services were equally likely to receive services in the last weeks of life as were HB or HC patients. Treatment-setting differences emerged, however, when comparing those who did not receive social service interventions until the last point of measurement. Only 15 percent of HB patients were first-time recipients of social services within a few weeks of death, compared to 40.9 percent of HC and 37.6 percent of CC patients. However, the number of new recipients at the last measure was so small among both hospice groups that these percentages were not significantly different.

Statistical models were developed to estimate the likelihood of receiving a social service intervention during three distinct time periods: the initial measure, throughout study duration, and the final measure prior to the patient's death. Figure 6.5 presents the estimates for each treatment setting over the three time periods. The estimated level of social service receipt was significantly higher in the HB and HC groups than among nonhospice patients over all three periods. The HB and HC estimates were nearly equal at all three points in time.

These comparisons are somewhat surprising if the reader expected there to be little or no social service use among nonhospice patients. Although all of these patients were identified and served in a medical setting, there was no effort made to identify settings with well-developed social service and support systems. Rather, as was described in chapter 3, nonhospice patients were identified via inpatient oncology units, outpatient clinics, and radiation therapy clinics in a diverse set of community and academic hospitals. The access to and delivery of social services to patients in such settings should reflect that which is provided to terminal oncology patients served in the better settings across the country. Despite the surprisingly high level of social service use among nonhospice patients, hospice patients were still more likely to receive such services at all points during the course of the study. The pattern of prehospice social service utilization clearly reflects a type of admission process that seldom is

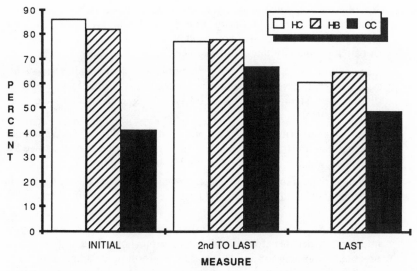

Figure 6.5   Estimated Receipt of Social Services by Time prior to Death

made available for CC patients. That hospice patients are more likely to receive social services in the last weeks of life presumably reflects the psychosocial values of the hospice movement.

Summary

This chapter has described the differences in the medical and social services patients receive in HB and HC hospices with those received by patients in the conventional-care systems. Conclusions as to whether exposure to the hospice system and philosophy of care caused the differences observed must be cautious, given possible self-selected differences in the patient populations. However, the evidence suggests that at least part of the differences can be reasonably attributed to the hospice-care modality. With this in mind, the findings can be summarized as follows:

- Conventional-care patients were more likely than hospital-based or home-care hospice patients to receive intensive medical interventions such as chemotherapy, radiation therapy, and surgery in the last and next-to-last weeks prior to death.
- CC patients receiving such intensive services at the initial measure were also significantly more likely than HB or HC patients to also have received them at the last measure prior to death.
- Conventional-care patients were more likely to receive diagnostic tests such as blood tests and X rays at every point prior to death.

- No differences among the three groups were observed in the likelihood of patients' receiving oxygen or respiratory therapy at any point during the study period. This overall comparison was confirmed by a special analysis of patients clinically likely to be in need of such services.

- Use of intravenous solutions and receipt of transfusions among patients with liver metastases and hemorrhages late in the terminal phase of their disease was significantly more likely among conventional-care than hospice patients.

- Analgesics prescribed for HB patients were more likely to have a regular specified administration schedule than to be prescribed on an as-needed basis than was the case for either the HC or CC group.

- Social service receipt was more prevalent among hospice patients throughout the study period and during the last weeks of life than among conventional-care patients.

- Finally, it appeared that the social service component of the hospice intervention began before hospice admission, possibly as a part of the process of applying for and being assessed for hospice admission.

7

The Last Weeks of Life: Does Hospice Care Make a Difference?

JOHN N. MORRIS,
SYLVIA SHERWOOD,
SUSAN M. WRIGHT,
AND CLAIRE E. GUTKIN

One of the most dreaded of diagnoses, cancer evokes a variety of strong fears. Among the images associated with cancer are those of severe and relentless pain, disfigurement, separation from friends and families, and loss of physical and mental functioning, social roles, and economic self-sufficiency (e.g., Cassel 1982; Cohen 1982; Turk and Rennert 1981; Bonica 1980; Lipman 1980; Bond 1979a; Chapman 1979; Stedeford 1979; Mitchell and Glicksman 1977; Maguire 1976; Graham et al. 1971; Holland 1973; Saunders 1967). Many still react to a cancer diagnosis as though to a death sentence, although there has been growing recognition that some forms of this multifaceted disease can be successfully treated.

Both the fear and the objective realities associated with cancer threaten the individual's quality of life. If the disease does proceed to its terminal phase, there are likely to be pervasive changes in activities, interpersonal relationships, physical status, and the rhythms and textures of daily life. Preserving as much as possible of the quality of life often takes precedence over length of survival.

Quality of life has emerged as a significant—some would say the most significant—criterion for terminal care. It is far from a simple criterion, however, either in its conceptualization or assessment. Much of this chapter is concerned with the specific methods utilized by the NHS for assessment of this key outcome. Although we employed what we judged to be adequate measures under the circumstances, we believe the search should continue for better ways to measure this complex concept.

The findings detailed in this chapter suggest that hospice care has some positive and no negative effects on cancer patients in their last weeks of life when compared with conventional medical care. In this sense, the hospice experiment seems to be working; those who have selected this option receive care at least as effective as do those who enter the traditional care system. Furthermore, in some—but not all—respects, quality of life appears to be superior for hospice patients. This pattern of results does not confirm hospice superiority in every facet of care, but does indicate that some of the most basic aims are being achieved, including the continuity of intimate social support. At the same time, hospice care did not result in the all-encompassing types of quality-of-life benefits over and above conventional care that many would have expected. In many respects, the outcomes of conventional care are comparable. Quality of life of patients choosing conventional care will not be appreciably different from what they would have been had they been exposed to hospice care.

The Quality of Life: Conceptualization and Measurement

Concerns of terminal-care cancer patients must be conceptualized from a holistic perspective. Positive outcomes include the prevention and alleviation of physical and psychological distress, maintenance of physical and mental functioning, and the involvement of a supportive network of informal relations. The literature suggests that these components of quality of life are strongly related and that interventions affecting one area also affect the others (Bloom 1982; Cohen 1982; Turk and Rennert 1981; Follick, Zitter, and Kulich, in press).

The area that has received most attention in the literature is "pain." Since the pioneering efforts of Dr. Cicely Saunders, important advances have been made in drug therapy (Lipman 1982, 1980; Walsh and Saunders 1981; Adriaensen, Mattelaer, and Van de Walle 1980; Twycross 1979; Symonds 1977; Saunders 1976). The common belief that pain is always a concomitant of cancer is unfounded (Lipman 1980). Studies reveal that, while the proportion is sometimes higher in the hospital setting, generally 50 percent or more of cancer patients do not suffer from severe pain; even in the terminal phase, a sizable number are reported to have little or no pain (Lipman 1980; Bond 1979a; Benoliel and Crowley 1974; Twycross 1984). Nevertheless, as is pointed out by Lipman (1980), "when that type of pain does occur it so envelops the patient's total existence that the pain becomes the focus of the existence. Patients in agony often do not retain their dignity. Caregivers and family members often cope poorly." Alleviating and managing the pain requires constant monitoring and is difficult (Benoliel and Crowley 1974).

Other negative physical effects of cancer are well recognized. Karnofsky's pioneering scale development work (Karnofsky et al. 1948; Karnofsky and Burchenal 1949) has resulted in the best-known function scale used in oncological research. The Karnofsky Performance Status measure and others like it emphasize physical functioning, but frequently symptoms such as nausea, diarrhea, shortness of breath, and anorexia that are carried by the disease process contribute to a reduction in functional capacity. As such, symptoms other than pain are also important targets of terminal-care interventions.

It has been hypothesized that cancer patients are at increased risk of depression and negative emotional states, although others have noted that this is related to physical deterioration (Cohen 1982; Weisman, Worden, and Sobel 1980; Bond 1979a; Gusterson 1977; Maguire 1976; Houston and Holmes 1974; Holland 1973). To the extent that patients' mood states are reflections of their quality of life, this, too, is an area that is germane for intervention. Indeed, the recent emphasis on the psychosocial status of oncology patients in the hospice and nonhospice systems lends support to the notion that this is an important area of outcome.

The importance of patient satisfaction with the formal network of care providers has also been noted (Bond 1979a; Chapman 1979). When patients are disappointed in their personal relationships with the physician, nurse, and other providers of care, they may be more likely to be uncooperative in their own treatment (Wolf et al. 1978; Davis 1971; Hayes-Bautista 1976; Kirscht 1977); this noncompliance in turn may have negative consequences on patients' quality of life.

Social contact and relations are also an important aspect of quality of life for the cancer patient. Social support includes instrumental assistance and affective relationships by and with significant others in the patient's informal network (Bloom 1982; Cohen 1982; Chapman 1979; Cassel 1976). Indeed, researchers have found that patients with more social support exhibit greater adjustment (Yalom 1977; Bloom, Ross, and Burnell 1978).

In summary, quality of life of the dying patient is multidimensional and must be conceptualized in terms of physical, emotional, and social domains, although there appears to be a complex potentiality unifying interrelationships among many of these domains. We identified a series of key quality-of-life outcome measures in each of these domains that we felt would be sensitive to change in a life span of only a few weeks. These are:

- pain and symptoms.
- functional status, physical and mental.
- emotional quality of life.
- social involvement with informal supporters.
- satisfaction with care.

We also considered patients' quality of life as a global construct. Building on the recent work of Spitzer and his associates (Spitzer et al. 1981), a number of summary indices were developed for health status, physical functioning, and the emotional-outlook components of quality of life. These can be considered as measures of overall quality of life.

Three practical issues were seen as crucial in evaluating the effect of hospice care. First, nearly one-quarter of the patients in the hospice sample died within fourteen days of intake into the program, and slightly over one-half had died within a six-week period. Obviously, to affect patients' lives, the hospice program must work quickly. Therefore, we felt it was important to assess the effect of length of "exposure" to the hospice program on the outcomes experienced by patients.

Second, we felt that measures of quality of life for terminal cancer patients had to be germane to their experience of life and sensitive to changes that might be caused by an intervention such as hospice care. For example, functional deficits were anticipated to be area-specific (e.g., patients no longer are capable of working at a job, but most would retain abilities in the areas of self-care and mobility). Pain and other symptoms were expected to be very salient when present but to vary considerably in prevalence. It was considered unlikely that significant numbers of patients would be found to be dissatisfied with the care they were receiving. Initial interviews supported all these assumptions: only 11 percent of the patients reported experiencing horrible or excruciating pain, 92 percent were neither working in any capacity nor managing their households, 50 percent had at least some independence in mobility, and 51 percent were in the highest two categories of the seven-level patient-satisfaction-with-care scale.

Third, we felt that the general social environment within which hospice care is implemented should be considered. Family and friends' involvement in providing care is an important aspect of the environment. If help from family and friends is substantial, the need for formal service intervention is reduced. In the most extreme case, the amount of informal support provided could obscure the impact of any services provided by other sources such as hospices. Indeed, 85 percent of all sample members had strong informal supports. About three-quarters received more than two hours of care on an average day from their principal care person (PCP), with as many as 60 percent receiving four or more hours and 40 percent receiving eight or more hours. Informal support and contacts with persons other than the PCP who did not live with the patient were also prevalent in our sample of terminal patients. Fully 70 percent of patients received an average of one or more hours of contact from nonhousehold family and friends on a daily basis. The levels of involvement are massive; they characterize both the hospice and conventional-care environments (the latter at a somewhat lower intensity level).

All of these factors were considered in both conceptualizing our analytic models and in interpreting the results. The section below describes the approach taken to analyze the quality-of-life (QL) data, specifically focusing upon certain issues particularly pertinent to the QL data gathered from patients and their PCPs.

The Analytic Approach

The Sample

The quality-of-life analyses were based on the follow-up sample. Selection of these patients was designed to make the samples as comparable as possible. (The specifications for this follow-up sample [Sample 4] are described in chapter 2.) Patients in hospice care and their families were interviewed *after* hospice admission. Therefore, no true measure of how the patient was faring *prior* to hospice exposure is available. In order to identify independent variables not affected by how long a patient had already been in a hospice at the time of his or her first interview, we examined the relationship between the outcome measures and the number of days between interview and hospice-program admission. Interestingly, a relationship between outcome and time (duration of exposure to hospice care) was only observed among patients interviewed *more* than seven days after hospice admission. Consequently, all QL analyses exclude those few individuals (less than 5 percent) who were not interviewed within seven days of entry into a hospice. Since there was no commensurate program admission date in the conventional-care sites, no exclusions were made on this basis.

Once the initial patient/PCP interview contact had occurred, an attempt was made to maintain a regular schedule of interview contacts. The first follow-up interview was scheduled to occur in seven days. The potential for sample loss was the main factor in choosing this time interval; a two-week interval would have excluded from the follow-up sample a large number of patients who died within two weeks of hospice admission. After this first one-week follow-up, a regular schedule of biweekly contacts was established and sustained until the patient died.

Patient data were gathered by interview at each of these contacts; an abbreviated version of the initial patient interview was utilized at each of the follow-up contacts. The instruments were designed to be administered in a brief period of time in order to minimize patient burden. We recognized that some patients would never be able to communicate with an interviewer and others would lose this ability as death approached. Therefore, some items in the patient interview were answered by proxy (i.e., the PCP) if the patient was unable to communicate. To assure a comparable data source for all patients, at each contact the interviewer rated the patient using the Karnofsky Performance Status Index (patient functioning) rating.

As will be recalled from chapter 2, all patients had to have a PCP. This individual had to be a family member or close friend and could specifically not be a health-care provider who might bias results. These principles were applied in selecting patients for all three samples. The PCP was the ideal source of information about the patient. The PCP always had a close relationship with the patient; over 50 percent were spouses, approximately 25 percent were children, and another 8 percent were siblings. Therefore, at each of the interview contacts, the PCP was asked to complete an assessment form providing information about the patient's functional status, health status, global quality-of-life services, and treatments received.

As noted in chapter 2, the patient-interview data were converted from a prospective flow of data from admission to death to a retrospective flow from the date of death back to that interview occurring within fourteen days of death to that occurring around fifteen weeks before death. Many patients died shortly after hospice admission or study entry, making it difficult to find a common analytic time frame for comparing the quality-of-life outcomes experienced by terminal cancer patients in hospice and nonhospice settings. We chose to compress the data closest to death and progress backward (e.g., starting at one week prior to death, going to three weeks prior to death, and so forth). Utilizing this strategy, most patients had an interview close to death, while fewer had outcome data as one moved backward in time. This approach controls for any differences in the proximity to death of the sample members being compared, a crucial consideration given the possibility that there might be underlying physical/psychological/social processes that could cause these patients to experience discrete shifts in quality of life as death approached. Physical deterioration, confusion, pain, and decreased social involvement were expected to become more prevalent in those who were closer to death.

Procedures Controlling for Sample Differences

Data from the initial patient/PCP interview were used to create separate adjustment equations for the regression procedures. The use of three equations for which estimates were made for the "average" hospice patient made it possible to phrase our research question as follows: What is the likely outcome were the "average hospice patient" to receive care under either of the two hospice modalities or in a conventional-care setting?

Correlations between one or more of our outcome measures and variables such as age, race, religion, marital status, living arrangement, social class, and so forth have also been reported in the literature (Bloom 1982; Dohrenwend and Dohrenwend 1981; Bond 1979b; Kessler 1979; Christensen 1978; Melzack 1974; Lilienfeld, Levin, and Kessler 1972). The array of potential independent variables used as adjusters in the regression equations was extensive; forty-nine separate items were ultimately used in one or more of the regression analyses for the array of dependent outcome variables under investigation. These variables can be broken down into eight groups, including: (1) descriptors and demographics; (2) help received; (3) burden on PCP; (4) patient pain and discomfort; (5) patient's medical condition, treatments, general health, and mobility; (6) patient's mental/emotional state; (7) quality-of-life assessments; and (8) length of program exposure and variables controlled by length of exposure.

The range of values for each of the forty-nine variables in all three samples is

Table 7.1 Independent Variables Entering Regression Equations

Variable	Category Range		Selected Category	Percentage in Selected Categories		
				HC	HB	CC
Patient age	1 21–44	5 75+	75+	11.4	10.0	2.9
Number children in hour's drive	0 None	3 3+	None	15.6	8.6	6.1
Importance of religion to patient	1 Very	3 Not Very	Very	22.0	18.2	14.3
Patient is protestant	0 No	1 Yes	Yes	52.9	36.2	43.9
Medicare—Part A	0 No	1 Yes	Yes	76.5	81.2	45.6
Disability insurance	1 Yes	2 No	Yes	13.0	9.3	22.2
Patient lives alone	0 No	1 Yes	Yes	5.4	15.4	16.0
PCP in household	1 Yes	2 No	Yes	91.4	80.4	74.6
PCP is spouse	0 No	1 Yes	Yes	60.0	52.2	53.1
Patient lives with spouse/other relative	0 No	1 Yes	Yes	90.2	82.8	80.5
Supportive family/friends	1 Agree	3 Disagree	Agree	83.6	84.0	84.8
Non-PCP informal network involvement	0 None	7 Many Hours	None	4.0	4.0	4.0
PCP reduced leisure activities	0 Yes	1 No	Yes	12.7	17.1	22.9
Family distress	0 Lowest	11 Highest	Lowest	4.2	5.7	8.9
Bone pain last two weeks	1 Yes	2 No	Yes	54.7	50.6	54.7
Pain control	0 Controlled	1 Uncontrolled	Uncontrolled	23.6	18.1	21.1
Pain status last week	1 Better	3 Worse	Worse	27.1	23.9	29.2
Sought pain relief past week	1 Yes	2 No	Yes	70.0	70.3	73.3
PCP assessment of Pt's pain	1 None	4 Persistent	Persistent	10.6	12.9	21.9
Discomfort in past week	1 None	4 Severe	Severe	9.0	7.7	13.3
Karnofsky (Collapsed)	1 Worst	5 Best	Less Than 5	85.7	86.4	93.4
Patient uses catheter	1 Yes	2 No	Yes	13.2	20.8	29.2
Patient uses I.V.	1 Yes	2 No	Yes	1.2	7.7	34.9
Patient uses oxygen	1 Yes	2 No	Yes	16.6	19.3	30.8
Brain involvement	0 No	1 Yes	Yes	16.9	16.0	18.3

(contd.)

Table 7.1 Independent Variables Entering Regression Equations (contd.)

Variable	Category Range		Selected Category	Percentage in Selected Categories		
				HC	HB	CC
Health	0 Poor	2 Good	Poor	63.0	67.2	61.6
Patient's mobility past week	0 Worst	2 Best	Worst	44.4	60.0	48.9
Functional assessment	1 Best	4 Worst	Best	14.6	10.7	18.0
Dry mouth past week	0 None	6 Severe	None	20.5	27.0	23.8
Patient has vomiting problem	0 No	1 Yes	Yes	36.2	39.3	39.6
Prostate/uterine cancer	1 No	2 Yes	Yes	11.8	9.6	6.2
PCP mentions Pt dying	1 Mention	2 Not Mention	Mention	72.5	74.0	60.2
Awareness past week	1 Fully Aware	3 Worst	Worst	48.3	50.4	54.3
Patient disorientation	1 None	3 Severe	None	56.5	60.6	58.6
Patient's outlook in past week	0 Confused	2 Positive	Worst	16.3	15.1	18.3
Depression index	1 None	3 Most	Most	46.8	53.8	56.2
Emotional quality of life	0 Lowest	14 Highest	12–14	26.5	21.9	28.4
Patient is coping	1 Agree	3 Disagree	Agree	87.0	79.5	70.1
Satisfied with professional help available	1 Agree	2 Ambiv./No	Ambiv./No	9.5	8.5	11.6
Feels blue	1 Not at All	3 A Lot	A Lot	14.5	15.9	24.9
Physical quality of life	0 Lowest	7 Highest	Best	9.8	8.3	19.6
HRCA QL	0 Worst	10 Best	8–10	3.5	2.1	6.5
Uniscale	0 Lowest	14 Highest	12–14	8.1	6.9	19.5
Missing Initial Self-Report Data	1 None	2 Some	None	65.1	60.6	65.0

116

presented in table 7.1. In addition to the demographic and disease characteristics, the samples are contrasted on the basis of their initial interview outcome measures. Demographically, these three patient samples are similar to the overall sample; nonhospice patients are younger, more likely to live alone, but are more likely to have children close by. Indeed, nearly 85 percent of all three groups agreed that there was a supportive network of family and friends. Nonhospice patients' PCPs did report greater family reduction of leisure-time activities due to the illness than was the case for the hospice patients' families, but an overall index of family disruption revealed relatively similar levels in all three groups at the time of study entry.

Pain of various types was similarly prevalent in all three groups at the outset, with over 70 percent of patients having sought pain relief in the week before the interview. It should be noted, however, that nonhospice patients were rated by their informal PCP to be in persistent pain and have severe symptoms more than was the case for the two hospice patient groups.

Consistent with the fact that even at study entry nonhospice patients were more likely to be in a hospital, they were more likely to be using I.V. care, oxygen, or catheters than was the case for hospice patients. Nonetheless, as we saw in chapter 2, the three groups are similar with respect to cancer type and the presence of different types of metastases.

Responses to psychosocial items also showed some interesting differences. Nonhospice patients were less likely to mention during the course of our interview that they were dying than was the case for the two hospice groups (60 percent versus 72 percent HC and 74 percent HB). Nonhospice patients' PCPs were less likely to agree that the patient was coping with his or her situation at the time of this initial interview than was the case for hospice patients' PCPs. Among the 65 percent of patients able to answer interview questions, nonhospice patients were more likely to report feeling blue "a lot" than was the case for either hospice group (25 percent versus 14 percent HC and 16 percent HB). Despite these psychological differences, nonhospice patients were actually rated to have better physical quality of life by their PCP than was the case for either hospice group.

As can be seen, the three groups were somewhat similar but also differed in important ways. This meant that our efforts to understand what difference hospice care made had to statistically take into consideration these preexisting differences before comparing outcomes.

Quality-of-Life (QL) Analyses

The presentation of the quality-of-life findings is ordered by outcome domain: pain and symptoms, summary indices of overall quality of life, specific indicators of overall quality of life, social involvement, and service satisfaction. Several domains have multiple measures, and each is presented separately.

The comparison of outcomes across the three settings is presented in a graphic format for the three measures closest to death (see figures 7.1 to 7.8). The same key is used for each figure. Solid lines represent hospital-based hospice patients, dashes represent home-care hospice patients, and alternating long and short dashes represent conventional-care patients. When differences were found to be statistically significant, additional analyses were performed to evaluate whether differential effects exist based on length of exposure to hospice care and the proximity of the patient to death. In general, these analyses did not reveal differential effects and are, therefore, discussed only when germane.

The Effect of Hospice Care on Pain and Symptoms

Two measures of pain are reported here. Both involve an assessment by the PCP of the pain experienced by the patient. Tables 7.2 and 7.3 present the Pain Index, which is composed of a PCP pain judgment as well as a measure of patient discomfort and a question regarding whether the patient's pain was controlled as well as possible. The second measure focuses solely on whether the patient was judged to have persistent pain and is essentially a dichotomized version of the PCP pain judgment showed in table 7.2. In addition to the pain measures, a symptom scale was constructed based on an array of six symptoms. The scale is

Table 7.2   Scoring of Pain Index: Patient and PCP Proxy Indication of Whether Pain Is Controlled as Well as Possible

	Yes, Controlled as Well as Possible			
PCP Judgment of Past Week Patient's Discomfort	Free of Pain	Occasional Pain	Frequent Pain	Persistent Pain
Symptom Free	0	0	1	1
Tolerable Symptoms	0	0	1	2
Frequent Symptoms	0	1	2	3
Severe Symptoms	0	1	3	3

	No, Not Controlled as Well as Possible			
PCP Judgment of Past Week Patient's Discomfort	Free of Pain	Occasional Pain	Frequent Pain	Persistent Pain
Symptom Free	0	1	1	2
Tolerable Symptoms	0	1	2	3
Frequent Symptoms	1	2	3	4
Severe Symptoms	1	2	4	4

Score Range for Pain Index
Free of Pain = 0
Highest Pain = 4

Table 7.3   Percentage Distribution for Pain for Entire Sample at an Average
of 5, 3, and 1 Week prior to Death

Score	Percentage Distribution		
	5 Weeks	3 Weeks	1 Week
0 (free of pain)	34.6	32.9	28.6
1	18.7	14.8	13.6
2	25.5	29.3	30.6
3	17.8	18.2	20.9
4 (highest pain)	3.4	4.7	6.3
Sample	Mean	Median	N
	1.37	1.33	642
	1.47	1.58	850
	1.63	1.75	1,023

a summary count of the number of those six symptoms the patient reported or
that were reported by the patient's PCP when the patient was unable to respond
(table 7.4).

It was recognized at the outset that some patients would not be able to report
on their own condition as death approached. Of the 1,087 patients in the combined samples, only 674 (62 percent) were able to respond on the self-report
measures. Those who could provide self-report information showed moderate
agreement with ratings made by their PCPs. The Melzack self-report item had
similar correlations with PCP judgment (.43) and the pain index (.45). Although the available comparisons between patient and PCP ratings of pain indi-

Table 7.4   Scoring of Symptom Scale (Number of the following symptoms that patient or
proxy reports patient is experiencing at any level from mild to unbearably severe: nausea, dry
mouth, constipation, dizziness, fever, short breath)

Score	Percentage Distribution for Symptom Scale Item for Entire Sample at an Average of 5, 3, and 1 Week prior to Death		
	5 Weeks	3 Weeks	1 Week
0 No Symptoms	7.9	4.5	3.3
1	16.6	12.9	13.2
2	24.6	25.8	23.8
3	23.0	24.8	23.0
4	15.5	17.6	15.0
5	8.2	9.1	10.7
6 Six Symptoms	4.3	5.3	11.0
Sample	Mean	Median	N
	2.6	2.5	634
	2.9	2.8	660
	3.1	2.9	927

cate some commonality, it is also clear that this relationship is not strong enough to substitute one source of rating for the other.

The self-report data included here are limited to information obtained at point of intake into the sample and at the first follow-up interview because there was a sharp decrease in the number of patients able to respond to the Melzack item just prior to death.

The symptom scale is composed of patient or proxy (often the PCP) reports of whether the following symptoms are being experienced by the patient: nausea, dry mouth, constipation, dizziness, fever, and short breath. Because of the inclusion of proxy as well as patient data, these items did not demonstrate the sample loss of the Melzack pain item and more closely resemble the pain judgments made by the PCP.

The equations developed to adjust for sample differences in comparing patients' outcomes included age, presence or absence of bone metastases (a very painful condition), and initial measures of health, functional status, and pain at time of admission to the study. The relationships observed are consistent with the literature and other more detailed analyses of these data (Morris, Mor et al. 1986). Older patients reported less pain, and those with bone metastases reported more pain. As one might imagine, whether patients were in pain at the time of study entry was the best predictor of pain in the last weeks of life.

Impact Findings

About five weeks prior to death, there was little difference in the average level of pain reported for patients in all three care settings. Most patients were below the midpoint (a score of 2 in a 0-to-4 range) of the pain index scale. As death approached, the pain level increased to some extent in the conventional-care and home-care samples. The mean level of the hospital-based patients, however, followed a different pattern (comparisons are shown in figure 7.1). Between five weeks and three weeks prior to death, the pain level actually decreased, but then began to rise. At five weeks prior to death, the estimated mean score for patients in hospital-based settings was significantly lower than would be the case were they served in either conventional-care or home-care hospices. However, the pain levels of the three groups on the pain index began to converge by the week prior to death, so that the differences between the hospital-based patients and the other two groups are not significantly different. Thus, the prevalence of pain tends to increase as death approaches in all settings, suggesting the need to intervene more aggressively with analgesics and other interventions.

Table 7.5, which presents the estimated percentage of patients in each group who were in severe pain at the last two measures prior to death, reveals a similar pattern. The proportion of patients in persistent pain increases in all settings, but did so least in the hospital-based hospice group. As estimated, 22 percent of

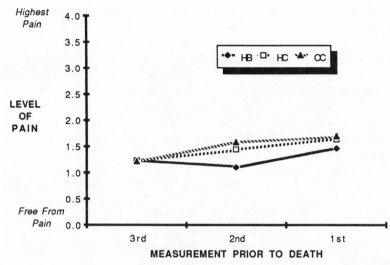

Figure 7.1   Mean Score on Pain Index for "Average" Hospice Patient as Death Approached

hospice-type patients would be in pain in a nonhospice setting. It should be emphasized that these estimates adjust for the preexisting differences between the groups on this measure. The prevalence of this type of persistent pain, uncontrolled with medication, in the nonhospice (as well as in the home-care hospice) group is consistent with the findings noted in the previous chapter regarding analgesic use. Hospital-based hospice patients had the highest level of analgesic use administered on a regular basis, and we see here that they were reported to have the lowest level of persistent pain.

The findings are also interesting in light of a study that compared dying

Table 7.5   Estimated Percent of Patients with "Persistent Severe Pain" on the PCP Pain Judgment as Death Is Approached Based on the Logistic Regression Analyses

	Second Measure prior to Death*	First Measure prior to Death
Home Care–Based Hospice	7	13
Hospital-Based Hospice	3	5
Conventional Care	14	22
Significant Difference at .05 Level or Lower		
Conventional Care versus Hospital-Based Hospice	—†	—†
Conventional Care versus Home Care–Based Hospice	ns	ns
Hospital-Based Hospice versus Home Care–Based Hospice	ns	ns

*No significant difference at this time period.
†Significant at the .05 level or lower.

cancer patients with specially designed home-care supportive services and dying persons cared for in a nursing home and in a hospital setting (Kassakian et al. 1979). The investigators reported that pain appeared to be less of a problem for the institutionalized than for patients cared for at home. They also noted some difficulty in pain management for patients at home due to patients and families not complying with the prescribed pain-control regimen. We found only slight differences in home-care hospice patients' pain and that reported by conventional-care patients. Hospital-based hospice care appeared to be superior to both alternatives with respect to pain management. Perhaps the observed differences are attributable to different factors. Home-care patients may have more pain because management protocols are more difficult to implement in a community as opposed to an inpatient hospice setting. On the other hand, nonhospice treatment-setting staff may have a different approach to and sensitivity toward patients' pain than is true for hospices. Indeed, numerous studies of analgesic prescription patterns reveal that traditional hospital staff underprescribe and are less likely to administer pain-control drugs prophylactically (Hardy and Pritchard 1977).

Studies of hospice staffing strongly point to the fact that a select group of health-care professionals choose to work in this area. Nonphysician hospice staff tend to be better educated, desire more autonomy, and invest more of their professional identity in their performance than is the case for hospital nurses (Greene 1984; Veatch and Tai 1980). Hospice staff may believe there is hope for the terminal patient, if only to achieve the goal of optimal pain control. This confidence may be further translated to the families and patients. In the nonhospice setting, where the usual goal and ethic of patient care is not palliation, the shift to the goal of comfort care, which can be quite complex, may be more difficult to make. This may result in a sentiment of helplessness being communicated to the patient, which, in turn, might exacerbate their sense of pain and hopelessness. Clearly, all these interpretations are subject to the caution that for many patients in the sample, we relied on proxy data from the PCP. How this might alter the relationships discussed is not known at present.

Sensitivity analyses were conducted to determine whether pain outcome as measured by the PCP pain index differed as a function of length of exposure to hospice care. Long-stay hospice patients were no more likely to have low or high pain than were short-stay patients. One interpretation of this finding is that hospices work quickly to put into place a pain-control program for patients. Our findings reveal that hospital-based hospices are effective in keeping down the number of patients entering the last weeks of life who are in severe pain.

Figure 7.2 presents comparative findings for the symptom scale. The relative positions of the mean scores for the average hospice patient remain constant at the three measurement points closest to death: conventional-care patients reveal the highest symptom score, hospital-based hospices present the lowest, and home-care hospices are between the other two groups. Significant

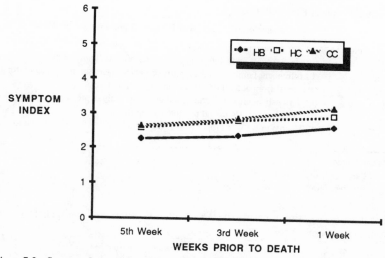

Figure 7.2   Symptom Index (Selected Measures Other than Pain) for "Average" Hospice Patient as Death Approached

differences were noted both at three weeks and one week prior to death. At three weeks, an average patient in a hospital-based hospice experienced fewer symptoms than would have been the case if served by either a conventional-care site or a home care–based hospice. At one week prior to death, this difference was statistically significant only in comparing the hospital-based hospice versus the conventional-care settings.

Sensitivity analyses of this outcome indicated that these findings held, regardless of level of exposure to hospice care and the number of symptoms patients reported at study entry.

The Effects of Hospice Care on Overall Quality of Life

This section describes the impact of hospice care on a variety of global indicators of patient quality of life. Interestingly, for these samples, there was little interrelationship between these measures and level of pain and symptoms. Overall quality of life was analyzed based on two summary indices. The first measure was derived from PCP responses to a series of questions about the patient's condition in various domains of functioning in the community (tables 7.6 and 7.7). The PCP was asked to categorize the patient's level of functioning in a series of separate areas. Responses to these five separate items were summed to yield the Hebrew Rehabilitation Center for Aged (HRCA) QL Index (a slight revision of the Spitzer Index [Morris, Suissa et al. 1986; Spitzer et al. 1981]), ranging from a low score of 0 to a high score of 10. The items form a reliable eleven-point summated scale (KR 20 Alpha Reliability = .65). The

Table 7.6   Scoring of HRCA QL Index

Item	Range of PCP Ratings of Patient's Status during Past Week
Daily Living	(0) Not managing personal care . . . (2) Self-reliant
Health	(0) Unconscious or feeling very ill . . . (2) Reports feeling great
Support	(0) Infrequent family/friend support, or patient unconscious . . . (2) Strong support from at least one family member/friend
Outlook	(0) Seriously confused or frightened or consistently depressed or unconscious . . . (2) Calm and positive; accepting
Mobility	(0) Unable to walk or propel wheelchair on own . . . (2) Usually able to walk

Score Range
Highest Possible Score = 10 (best)
Lowest Possible Score = 0 (worst)

Table 7.7   Percentage Distribution for HRCA QL for Entire Sample at an Average of 5, 3, and 1 Week prior to Death

	Percentage Distribution		
Score	5 Weeks	3 Weeks	1 Week
0 Worst	1.2	1.5	3.1
1	2.0	5.1	7.6
2	10.9	13.1	26.2
3	20.1	23.1	26.3
4	21.1	21.6	20.3
5	18.3	16.9	8.7
6	13.0	10.9	5.8
7	8.3	4.7	1.0
8	3.0	2.0	0.8
9	2.0	0.9	0.1
10 Best	0.2	0.2	0.2
Sample	Mean	Median	N
	4.40	2.50	662
	3.96	3.83	865
	3.14	3.00	1,046

five HRCA QL items include measures of patients' functioning and daily living activities, health status, social supports, emotional outlook, and mobility.

As patients deteriorate, measures such as the HRCA QL are characterized by considerable negative change in the last three weeks of life. Consequently, we felt that it was reasonable to believe that effects might be observed in these areas if hospice care was able to maintain patients' functioning as long as possible.

Figure 7.3 presents the results of comparing the three samples on the HRCA QL Index. There were no significant differences across the three samples at any of the time periods. The plot of the means over the five-week period suggests that a decrease in overall quality of life was occurring comparably across samples and was most accentuated just prior to death.

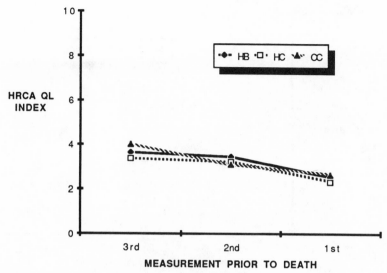

Figure 7.3   Mean Score on HRCA Quality-of-Life Index for "Average" Hospice Patient as Death Approached

In addition to this overall measure of quality of life, three more specific indicators were examined: the Karnofsky performance index, a measure of emotional quality of life, and an assessment of patient awareness. These measures, unlike the more general overall indices, specifically addressed the individual's physical and emotional responses as death was approached.

The Karnofsky Performance Status (KPS) was scored on the basis of observations of the patient made by the interviewer and was completed regardless of whether the patient was capable of being interviewed. NHS interviewers had been trained in making these judgments prior to the start of data gathering. All reached an acceptable level of reliability, and their judgments were shown to have strong predictive validity (Mor et al. 1984). The KPS is a ten-point rating scale, ranging from normal functioning (a score of 100) to moribund (10). The majority of individuals had scores in the range of 20 to 40 at all measurement points during their participation in this study. PCPs provided information concerning patients' emotional quality of life and level of awareness. The PCP chose one of four awareness categories, 1 being full range of mental faculties, and 4 indicating severe confusion. Emotional QL was measured using a visual analogue on which the PCP marked the spot on a continuum between two extremes indicating where the patient stood. It should be noted that the relationship of the PCP to the patient did not appear to influence the rating and therefore was not introduced into the regression equations. Findings for these three indices were virtually identical to those previously described for the overall quality-of-life measure.

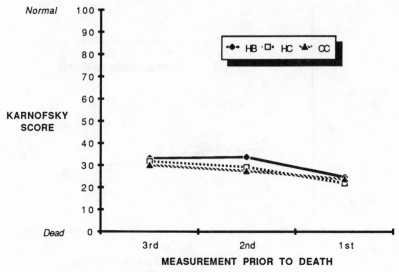

Figure 7.4   Mean Score on Karnofsky for "Average" Hospice Patient as Death Approached

Figures 7.4 and 7.5 present the results of comparing the Karnofsky Performance Status and the awareness measure. In these as well as the emotional quality-of-life scale, there were no significant differences across the three service modalities, even though there was a substantial decrease in quality of life in these measures as death approached. Thus, the hospice interventions did not

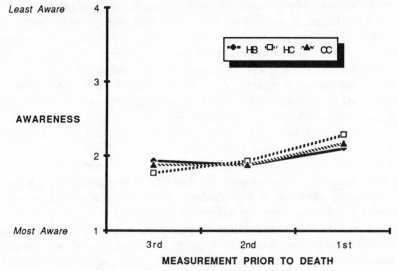

Figure 7.5   Mean Score on Awareness for "Average" Hospice Patient as Death Approached

alter the quality of life of terminal cancer patients in either the physical or emotional arenas as rated by PCPs.

The Effects of Hospice Care on Social Involvement

Four measures of patients' involvement in social activities were identified for the study: social involvement with family and friends other than the PCP, chatting with the PCP, the number of hours of direct care provided by the PCP, and an overall indicator of social quality of life.

The terminal-care patients included in the NHS sample were characterized by extensive informal support resources. Our analyses examined differences in social involvement during the last five weeks of life. As patients' needs increased, we expected to be able to see differences in how families spent time with patients. The inclusion of four separate measures of social involvement reflects the complex nature of social involvement for patients during the terminal phase of life. For example, patients residing in their own homes will depend more upon family and friends to meet their personal-care needs than will patients in an inpatient setting. On the other hand, hospitalized patients may be viewed as needing more social visiting than is the case for home-care patients. Based on expectations of this type, we hypothesized that sample comparison results would vary depending upon the social involvement indicator being evaluated.

The non-PCP informal network involvement index assessed the supportive and visiting activities by persons other than the PCP. At each interview, the PCP was asked to indicate the number of days in the previous two weeks during which family and friends performed direct caregiving activities as well as social visiting activities. The PCP also reported the number of hours per day in which each of these activities occurred during that two-week period of time. The resulting total of hours per day was then categorized into eight levels (see table 7.8). There were two measures involving PCP support and attention provided to the patient. One, the PCP instrumental support index, measures the number of hours of direct care provided solely by the PCP during the preceding two-week period. This, too, was categorized using the intervals seen in table 7.8. The second measure, chatting with household members (including the PCP), indicates time chatting with the patient during the preceding two-week period, measured as none, some, and a lot.

Social involvement was also measured as an overall estimate of social quality of life. The PCP rated the patient's overall social quality of life along a continuum where the two polar categories were fully described. At one extreme were persons with unsatisfactory relationships, characterized by being of poor quality and fewer in number; at the other extreme were persons with very satisfactory and extensive social relationships.

As expected, over the last five weeks of life there were significant dif-

Table 7.8   Scoring and Percentage Distribution of Non-PCP Informal Network Involvement
over a Two-Week Period for Entire Sample at an Average of 5, 3, and 1 Week prior to Death

Score	Percentage Distribution		
	5 Weeks	3 Weeks	1 Week
0 (Least) None	4.0	2.4	3.1
1 1–13 hours	27.8	27.2	25.4
2 14–28 hours	24.7	24.5	24.8
3 29–56 hours	18.2	17.7	17.0
4 57–112 hours	14.6	15.0	14.8
5 113–224 hours	7.2	10.4	11.1
6 225–448 hours	3.4	2.4	3.4
7 (Most) Over 449 hours	0.0	0.5	0.5
Sample	Mean	Median	N
	2.47	2.24	669
	2.59	2.33	882
	2.64	2.37	1,040

Note: Scoring and percentage distribution computed from number of days in last two weeks
patient received direct help or care from other (non-PCP) family or friends multiplied by the total
average hours of help provided on those days; plus number of days in last two weeks other (non-
PCP) family or friends visited patient multiplied by the total average hours visiting on those days

ferences among the groups on these measures. In general, the patients in home-
care hospices fared significantly better than would have been the case in a
conventional-care setting. This applies particularly to two measures: the non-
PCP informal involvement index, and the hours of help by the PCP. Figure 7.6
presents the comparison of PCP direct-care hours per patient day by treatment
setting. As can be seen, hospice patients in home-care settings consistently
received more support than was the case for patients in either of the inpatient-
based programs. When contact with other than the PCP was examined, only the
HC-versus-CC differences were significant, and even these were substantially
smaller than for the PCP direct-care measure. Hospital-based hospices were in
between the levels of support found for home-care and nonhospice settings.
The high level of PCP support observed for home-care hospice patients was
what probably made it possible for these patients to remain at home. The
important role of the PCP, over and above support provided by nonhousehold
family members, is highlighted by these findings. Need for family support is
highest in the home-care group, and, clearly, the PCP is meeting most of that
need.

A measure of overall social quality of life was assessed and compared across
groups (fig. 7.7). In all three samples, the average scores at all three measurement points were high. The means for the two hospice groups were very similar
but tended to be somewhat lower than those of the conventional-care sample.
The comparison between the conventional-care sample and the other two
groups was statistically significant at the measure closest to death but not at the

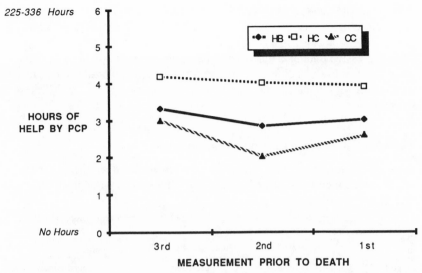

Figure 7.6   Mean Score on Hours of Help by PCP for "Average" Hospice Patient as Death Approached

earlier points. As noted, these differences are small, and all three patient groups were rated as having very high social quality of life. In cases where there is so little room for improvement, the meaningfulness of statistically significant differences can be questioned. This is particularly true since the amount of

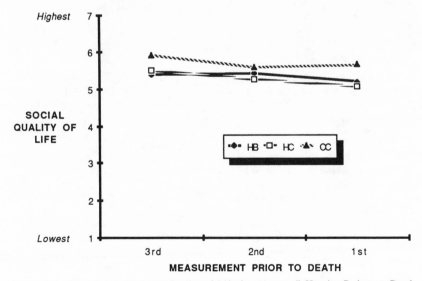

Figure 7.7   Mean Score on Social Quality of Life for "Average" Hospice Patient as Death Approached

direct care and chatting observed for conventional-care patients was significantly lower than was the case for the two hospice samples. What meaning, then, should be attached to this observed difference in social quality of life? The most impressive finding is that hospice patients received high levels of social support. The observed differences in overall social quality of life were rather small, so in all likelihood, the higher overall rating by nonhospice PCPs is a spurious finding.

The Effects of Hospice Care on Satisfaction with Care

Most patients reported being satisfied with the care received throughout the last five weeks of their lives (see table 7.9). This finding was based upon patient

Table 7.9 Percentage Distribution for Patient Service Satisfaction for Entire Sample at Initial Interview, First Follow-up, and Second Follow-up

	Percentage Distribution		
Score	Initial Interview	First Follow-up	Second Follow-up
0	3.5	2.5	1.2
1	3.5	3.4	3.7
2	8.6	8.1	6.4
3	14.4	14.6	13.0
4	19.0	18.0	16.6
5	24.8	25.1	24.2
6	26.2	28.4	35.0
Sample	Mean	Median	N
	4.21	4.54	778
	4.31	4.64	529
	4.53	4.88	409

Note: patient was instructed

I will read you some statements about the doctors, nurses, and others who may be caring for you. For each of these statements, tell me how you now feel using one of these responses:
  Agree
  Ambivalent
  Disagree
The DOCTOR tells me all I want to know about my illness.
The DOCTOR gives me a chance to say what is really on my mind.
It is hard to believe everything my DOCTOR tells me about my illness. (Scoring reversed on this item.)
I have doubts as to whether I am receiving the best care possible. (Scoring reversed on this item.)
I feel that my medical treatment was unnecessarily harsh. (Scoring reversed on this item.)
Decisions about my care seem to take an excessive amount of time. (Scoring reversed on this item.)
Coding:
  1 = Agree
  0 = Ambivalent/Disagree

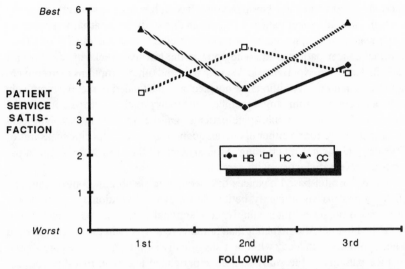

Figure 7.8   Mean Score on Patient Service Satisfaction for "Average" Hospice Patient after Intake

self-report. A sufficiently high percentage of patients was able to provide
ratings at intake and subsequent measuring points to allow for a straightforward
prospective analysis. As can be seen in figure 7.8, most patients reported being
satisfied over all three measurement periods. Despite the observed differences
between the three patient samples, the variation and relatively small sample
sizes made it unlikely that a statistically significant difference would be detected. The substantial fluctuations from measure to measure in all samples
suggest that the scores themselves are unstable, perhaps reflecting different
samples of patients measured or fluctuations in patients' perceptions of satisfaction with their care.

The important lesson from this finding appears to be that patients are fairly
satisfied with the medical and nursing care they receive, regardless of the
setting that cared for them. It may be that patients are satisfied with the choices
they made in selecting their model of care. Alternately, terminal cancer patients
are as generically satisfied with health-care providers as are all patients. In the
face of this global satisfaction, even if hospice patients were more satisfied it
would be very hard to prove it. In our view, then, a preferable interpretation is
that hospice care did not yield any reductions in patient satisfaction in the face
of a very different pattern of care.

Conclusions

While not all of the positive effects expected by hospice proponents were
found, some were. Most importantly, it does not appear that the hospice inter-

vention, whether hospital-based or home-based, has any negative effects on the lives of terminal cancer patients. Data from this study only partially support the hypothesis that hospice care has a positive effect upon the quality of life of terminal cancer patients. At some point in the last five weeks of life, hospice patients tended to experience less severe pain and other symptoms than conventional-care patients. Additionally, hospice patients tended to receive more help and social contact from family members and their principal care persons (PCPs) than was the case for nonhospice patients. On the other hand, no significant differences were found either in overall quality of life or in specific measures of physical and mental functioning. Similarly, no differences were found in patient-reported satisfaction with care.

It was hospital-based hospices that seemed to be able to control pain and other symptoms significantly better than either conventional care or home care–based hospices. Interestingly, conventional care, with its greater use of the acute hospital, did no better than home-care hospices in managing pain and other symptoms. Indeed, while not statistically significant, home care–based hospice patients in the study sample experienced less pain than the conventional-care patients. Significant differences to the benefit of hospital-based hospices in the proportion of patients reporting severe pain were sustained at the last measure, suggesting that the inpatient hospice was best able to manage pain at a time when it was most prevalent in other settings.

All patients had frequent social contact and received considerable direct care. Consistent with where patients spend their time, PCPs provided significantly more hours of help to patients in home care–based hospices than did PCPs of clients in hospital-based hospices or in conventional care. No differences were found, however, between conventional care and hospital-based hospices in this regard. Home care–based hospice patients also had significantly greater contacts than the conventional-care patients. The social quality-of-life assessments were high for all three groups at the three measurement points prior to death.

In summary, home-care hospice patients used the most informal care. Although the hospital-based model appears to surpass the home-care hospice model in pain control, a modified approach to monitoring the patient's pain level might improve the outcome for the home care–based patients. Even without such improvement, the home care–based hospice patients fared no worse than those in conventional care in controlling pain, and did so at a considerably lower cost (see chapters 4 and 5). From this perspective at least, the home-care hospice can be considered an effective and less costly treatment option for dying patients who prefer to spend their last weeks of life in their own homes.

8

The Effect of Hospice Care
on Where Patients Die

VINCENT MOR, JOHN N. MORRIS,
JEFFREY HIRIS,
AND SYLVIA SHERWOOD

"What does hospice care do?"

"Help dying people stay at home with their families."

This perception of hospice care appears to be dominant in the United States (Stoddard 1978; Buckingham and Lack 1978) although less so in England and Canada. Evidence that hospice care is fulfilling its promise might be sought, then, by answering two related questions: (1) Are terminally ill patients who are receiving hospice care more likely to die at home? and (2) Is this outcome perceived as satisfactory? It is possible, for example, that the desired goal (home death) might not be as highly valued when it actually happens, or that terminal care in an institutional setting might not prove as negative an experience as had been feared. Only appropriate research can answer such questions.

It should be noted immediately that home death actually is but one of many possible measures of hospice effectiveness. Palliation of symptoms, for example, is generally regarded by hospice organizations as a high-priority goal, independent of the site of death. Nevertheless, an evaluation of hospice care in the United States must necessarily include attention to the site of death and its correlates.

The hospice's emphasis upon care in the home is in sharp contrast to the prevailing norm with respect to the site of death in the United States. Perhaps this emphasis arose as part of a generalized societal reaction against the primacy of technological medicine and the hospital as its institutional repository (Cassel 1982). Recently, a special analysis conducted by the National Center for Health Statistics revealed that only 13.7 percent of people whose deaths were attributed to cancer died at home in 1979. Data from Cleveland reveal that there has been a shift in the period from 1957, when 30 percent of all cancer deaths occurred at home, to 1979, when only 15 percent of cancer deaths occurred at home. But if there was a trend toward death in a medical setting among cancer patients over the past three decades, there are signs that that trend may be reversing, perhaps as a direct result of the hospice movement.

Mor and Hiris (1983) summarized data from a number of hospice sources, noting that the proportion of cancer deaths at home per annum had been increasing in several upstate New York counties and townships west of Boston. The rate of change in these trends toward death at home appears to be related to the presence of hospices in the area. Both the hospice philosophy and the HCFA-supported demonstration project attempt to provide the maximum opportunity for terminally ill people to remain at home if this is their preference. Home nursing and other supportive services are made available for this purpose.

This chapter compares the site of death of patients served in hospices and conventional-care settings. Since home death per se is not necessarily a universally desirable outcome of hospice care, comparisons are also made of the values placed on where patients die and how long they were at home in their last days of life. Finally, we examine the factors that are associated with whether death occurs at home or in a medical setting.

Previous analyses of the population of hospice cancer admissions to demonstration hospices (Mor and Hiris 1983) revealed marked differences in the proportion of patients dying at home as a function of the type of hospice in which they were enrolled. However, limited patient-mix data were available for these analyses, particularly regarding patients' functioning and social-support availability. The analyses described in this chapter are based upon the richer set of data available for the follow-up sample of patients.

Methods

Two different samples are used to perform the analyses reported in this chapter. The first includes all patients in the follow-up sample for whom site of death was ascertained. The second is comprised of a subset of PCPs interviewed between 90 and 120 days after the death of the patient. This sample of PCPs is described in greater detail in the next chapter, on family outcomes. As will be recalled from the description of the hospice and comparison samples in chapter 2, all patients had homes in the community to which they could return following hospitalization episodes. This differs considerably from the traditional long-term-care patient population, many of whom reside permanently in nursing homes; none of our sample patients were like this.

Data for these analyses were derived from interviews, medical records, and hospice records.

Study discharge records were used to ascertain where the patient died. In general, this information came from hospice patient records, but frequently it was known only by the NHS interviewer. The latter was always the source of information about site of death in the conventional-care sample. Site of death was not known for 5.5 percent of the follow-up sample of patients.

Initial interviews with patient and PCP contained data for many of the independent variables regarding level of informal support available, patient's condition at study entry, and other patient and PCP background characteristics. The bereavement interview with the PCP included data pertaining to the PCP's satisfaction with where the patient died and his or her judgment of whether or not the patient had remained at home as long as he or she wanted to prior to death.

Three dependent variables were constructed and analyzed in this chapter. *Home death* is defined as "yes" if death occurred at home, or as "no" if in an inpatient hospice, an acute hospital, or a nursing home. *PCP satisfaction with where patient died* is defined on the basis of a single question asked of the PCP in the bereavement interview. The question was asked within the context of a series of items related to "regrets" the PCP had regarding the mode of treatment the patient experienced in his or her final months. Whether the *patient remained at home as long as he or she wanted* is also based upon a question asked of the PCP during the bereavement interview. The question was asked following a series of questions in which the PCP described the patient's last days.

Each of these three variables is treated as a separate dependent variable in this chapter. Additionally, we examined a composite measure of the congruence between where the patient actually died and where the PCP would have liked the patient to die. This further level of analysis contributes to our understanding of the social value associated with home death.

The Analytic Approach

The analysis was carried out in two stages. The first involved developing a listing of domains and measures thought to be associated with patients' and families' choice of site of death and the other dependent variables. Little literature was available to guide us in this process. Consequently, we related to home death a broad array of independent variables that characterized both the patient and the PCP. The next stage involved the development and refinement of a multivariate logistic regression model to predict the dependent variable among the three different groups of patients using those variables found to be related to home death. Procedures similar to those outlined in chapter 2 were employed. The predicted site of death of an "average" demonstration hospice patient was ascertained in each of the three equations, thus estimating the unique impact of treatment setting on site of death.

Findings

The Site of Death among Hospice and Nonhospice Patients

Dying at home was a frequent outcome for patients in the HC setting (62.5 percent). Those receiving care in HB settings were more than twice as likely to die at home than were conventional-care patients (27.2 percent to 12.7 percent). This pattern of findings indicates that the hospice alternative does tend to meet one of the goals for which it has been designed: the opportunity to live one's last moments at home. The difference in percentage of home deaths between the two types of hospice organizations, however, is an appreciable one, presumably attributable to different practices and a somewhat different mix of patients served.

The percentage of CC cancer patients dying at home in our study is similar to the national average from the 1979 final mortality statistics (National Center for Health Statistics 1982). The percentage of HC follow-up patients dying at home is almost identical with that of *all* HC patients admitted, regardless of whether they became part of the follow-up sample (see chapter 2). However, the percentage of HB follow-up sample patients dying at home is somewhat higher than for the *population* of HB admissions. [1]

Adjusted Estimates of the Home Death Rate by Setting

In this section we present the findings of the multivariate analyses of site of death among patients in each treatment setting, adjusting for the mix of patients in each of the three samples. To estimate the probability of a patient's dying at home had he or she been served in either an HC, an HB, or a CC setting, we constructed a logistic regression equation for each sample using independent variables that were conceptually relevant and empirically predictive of home death. The "average" patient served in a demonstration hospice was then "passed through" each equation in order to estimate his or her probability of home death.

Had the average hospice patient been served in a CC setting, he or she would have had a probability of .24 of dying at home. Contrasting this value with the unadjusted rates presented above reveals that the equation substantially adjusted the actual value. The average patient in an HB setting had a .39 probability of home death, while in an HC setting the probability was .53. Despite the drop in the proportion of HC home deaths, patients in an HC setting are still

---

1. The difference between the home death rate among HB *follow-up* sample members and the population of HB admissions (see chapter 2, table 2.4) is largely attributable to an underrepresentation of very short-stay patients who were admitted into the hospice inpatient unit and who died there. These patients were not able to be contacted for inclusion in the follow-up sample, given their short survival after admission.

Table 8.1   Percent of Patients in Each Treatment Setting with a Given Attribute Who Died at Home

	HC	HB	CC
Base Rate of Home Death	62.5	27.2	12.7
Demographic			
Patient is female	61.8	28.8	14.9
Patient is single, divorced, separated	52.5†	24.9	17.1
PCP is patient's spouse	64.0	27.1	11.6
PCP is patient's child	63.6	27.2	5.1*
Patient's age is over 54	62.9	26.9	12.6
Patient's age is over 74	68.2*	23.1	18.2
Patient is Jewish	49.2†	22.9	25.8
Patient is Catholic	64.0	29.8	15.0
PCP age is over 54	62.9	26.3	16.0
PCP age is over 74	70.4*	24.6	17.7
Social			
Patient lives alone	39.4‡	19.2	4.6
PCP lives in patient's household	63.6	29.9	14.1
Patient wants last 3 days at home	62.0	40.8†	27.2*
Medical			
Karnofsky Performance Status is less than 30	72.4*	26.1	5.8*
Patient is catheterized	68.1	26.4	7.8
Patient is in active therapy	50.6†	32.9	9.3
Patient has very bad pain	58.7	27.9	6.9*
Patient not hospitalized in last month	64.5	31.4	29.5‡
Patient awareness unimpaired	57.0†	29.1	14.3
Patient does not manage activities of daily living (ADL)	67.2‡	27.9	11.6
Patient received "intensive" medical therapy	56.7*	28.8	12.0

*Significant at the .05 or beyond.
†Significant at the .01 or beyond.
‡Significant at the .001 or beyond.

significantly more likely to die at home than in either an HB ($p < .01$) or a CC ($p < .001$) setting. Patients served in an HB setting are also significantly ($p < .01$) more likely to die at home than are patients served in a CC setting.

Factors Affecting Home Death

A broad array of demographic, medical, functional, social-support, and psychological variables was examined for their relationship to home death. The proportion of patients in each sample with a given characteristic is listed in table 8.1. Whether home death is more or less likely in comparison with the average decedent from that setting is indicated by an asterisk. Both the number and direction of variables significantly related to home death differed across treatment settings. For example, nonhospice patients with a low Karnofsky Performance Status score were less likely to die at home than those with a higher KPS score. Among HC patients, this relationship was reversed; patients with a low KPS were more likely to have died at home. The description that follows is presented within sample type, focusing upon those patient and family characteristics that were found to be related to home death.

Home care–based hospice patients *more* likely to die at home include:

- those who were married.
- patients *not* living alone.
- patients admitted in poor functional condition.
- patients not in active therapy at the time of hospice admission.
- patients over the age of seventy-four.
- patients whose awareness was impaired at time of hospice admission.

Factors influencing home death in the HB population include:

- among patients able to respond to the initial interview, those who said they want to spend their last three days at home.

Within the CC sample, patients *more* likely to have died at home include:

- patients whose PCP was *not* a child.
- patients entering the study with some residual functioning.
- patients *not* in a lot of pain at study entry.
- patients *not* hospitalized in the month before study entry.
- patients wanting to spend their last three days of life at home.

It can be seen that factors associated with where a patient died were not comparable across the three settings. For example, single, divorced, or separated patients in the HC setting were significantly less likely to die at home than was the case for similar persons served by HB hospices or in a nonhospice setting. When a factor was significantly related to home death in more than one setting, it did not necessarily have the same meaning. For example, poor functional status at time of admission was related to home death among HC patients but to hospital death among nonhospice patients. On the other hand, patients wishing to spend their last three days of life at home were more likely to die at home in two settings (HB and CC) but not in an HC setting. This latter finding may arise because the actual percentage of persons dying at home is highest in the HC group, suggesting that the saliency of the desire to die at home is stronger when the care setting is not predisposed to support death at home.

The description above focused upon the major demographic, social-support, and medical factors associated with home death. Clearly, other factors that are not necessarily characteristics of the patient and his or her family were related to home death. Home death presumably reflects a complex of forces that shape the intermediate and final decisions of patients, their families, and their providers of care. The condition of the patient and where he or she was at the time of study entry is presumably influenced by prior decisions and as such serve as a proxy for the "path" taken. We examined the relationship between home death and where the patients were at the time of study entry. We found that where the patient was when he or she entered the study (i.e., either in an inpatient setting or at home) has a major influence upon where he or she dies in all three samples. Of the minority of nonhospice patients (31 percent) initially seen at home, 24.7 percent died at home. Only 7.7 percent of nonhospice patients initially interviewed in an institution died at home. For the HB sample, 45 percent of those interviewed at home died at home. Only 12.3 percent of the HB sample initially interviewed in an inpatient setting died at home. HC sample patients were rarely in an inpatient setting upon study entry; however, being in an inpatient setting at the outset was also predictive of dying in a medical setting. Clearly, current location was a powerful predictor of final location.

A Multivariate View of Factors Affecting Home Death

To improve our understanding of characteristics that affect home death when other factors are controlled, table 8.2 presents the independent variables used in

Table 8.2   Logistic Regression Equations Predicting Home Death for Each Care Setting

	Regression Coefficients		
Independent Variables	Home-Care Hospice	Hospital-Based Hospice	Conventional Care
Survival after study admission (days)	−.106	.223	.509
Initial interview at home (1 = yes)	2.769‡	1.910‡	.697
Patient lives alone (1 = yes)	−.584	−.054	−1.22
Family income (categories) (0 = Low; 3 = High)	.242‡	.072	−.035
Patient over age 74 (1 = yes)	.436	−.454	1.01
Patient is Jewish (1 = yes)	−.879‡	−.125	1.184
Patient is Catholic (1 = yes)	−.117	.153	.439
Karnofsky Performance Status under 30 at admission (adm.) (1 = yes)	.779†	−.245	.058
Patient pain/discomfort at adm. (hi = severe)	−.048	−.166	−.200
Not hospitalized month before study adm. (1 = yes)	.132	−.624*	.764
Patient awareness unimpaired at adm. (1 = yes)	−.374*	−.576*	−.420

*Significance level of .05 or beyond.
†Significance level of .01 or beyond.
‡Significance level of .001 or beyond.

the logistic regression equations and their associated regression coefficients. The relative importance of each variable is indicated by its level of significance in the equation. Controlling for a number of factors simultaneously can be useful in identifying which factor has the strongest relationship with the dependent variable. As we have seen, one of the more important determinants of home death in both the HB and HC equations is where the patient was when he or she entered the study. Controlling for a host of other factors, those entering from an inpatient setting were less likely to die at home. Patients' awareness upon study entry was significantly related to death *not* occurring at home for both the HB and HC groups. In the HC equation, patients with poor functional status upon admission were more likely to die at home even when survival beyond the initial interview is controlled. In the HC equation, demographic factors such as family income and being Jewish were also related to home death. As noted earlier, patient-report variables from the initial interview such as mood state and expressed wishes regarding the last three days of their lives were also found to be related to home death. However, as we noted in chapter 7, a substantial proportion of patients were unable to respond to interview questions even at the first interview. Consequently, inclusion of these variables in a model predicting site of death would have reduced the number of patients in the analysis and biased the results to a nonrandom selection process.

Overall, demographic and patient characteristic factors proved to have rather little differential relationship to the likelihood of home death. The summary of patient characteristics provided in table 8.3 indicates that fifteen of the twenty-one variables showed no relationship to site of death. Living with the PCP and receiving services in the home were among the few variables related to likelihood of home death. Most interesting, perhaps, among the nondifferences are the variables describing the condition of the PCP following the death of the patient. PCPs who cared for patients with home deaths did not appear any more vulnerable to negative personal outcomes than did those who cared for a person who died in an inpatient setting. Indeed, in some cases, the relationships go in the opposite direction, suggesting that PCPs who had physical difficulties, suicidal thoughts, or alcohol problems were probably predisposed to these manifestations of stress regardless of what setting of care had been provided. It is also of some interest that biological factors (cancer type and organ involvement) also were not related to site of death. The tentative conclusion arising from the findings presented in table 8.3 is to underscore the importance of the availability of support in the home as a precondition to enabling terminally ill patients to remain home as long as possible. Apparently, the philosophy of a hospice also enables those who want to die at home to do so.

Table 8.3 Likelihood of Home Death by Site Type and Patient Characteristics

Patient Characteristics	HC	HB	CC
Age	NS	NS	Old More Likely*
Patient in therapy at study intake	NS	NS	NS
Free from pain in last 3 days, based on PCP at bereavement interview	NS	NS	NS
Patient home as long as wanted, based on PCP at bereavement interview	True More Likely‡	True More Likely‡	True More Likely‡
PCP encouraged patient to take therapy; wish hadn't—Bereavement interview	NS	NS	NS
PCP takes medications (meds) for nerves at bereavement interview	NS	NS	Take Meds Less Likely†
PCP increases alcohol	NS	NS	NS
PCP thinks of suicide	NS	NS	NS
PCP strapped financially while patient alive	NS	NS	NS
PCP can't respond to others' needs when patient alive	NS	NS	NS
Patient lives with PCP	NS	Yes More Likely‡	Yes More Likely* (.06)
Health limit PCP	NS	NS	NS
PCP's life complicated by other crises at study entry	NS	NS	NS
Patient sex	NS	NS	NS
Patient discomfort at study entry	NS	Less Discomfort More Likely*	NS
PCP employed full-time at study entry	NS	NS	NS
PCP education	NS	NS	NS
Patient income	NS	NS	High More Likely*
PCP reduced work because of patient care	NS	NS	NS
Cancer type and/or organ system involvement	NS	NS	NS
Number of M.D. visits since patient died—Bereavement interview	NS	NS	NS

NS = Nonsignificant.
* Significant at .05.
† Significant at .01.
‡ Significant at .001.
→ Direction of relationship to home is noted when it is significant.

Satisfaction of PCPs with Patients' Site of Death

The previous discussion highlighted the role of hospice care in altering residential decisions during the last days of life. This section describes the values associated with death at home.

Most PCPs (85.9 percent) report being satisfied with where the patient died (table 8.4). Satisfaction is highest when the patient died at home (93.9 percent of the PCPs) or in an inpatient hospice setting (88.7 percent of the PCPs). Among patients who died in an acute hospital or other inpatient setting, a substantially larger percentage of PCPs was dissatisfied with where the patient died (24.4 percent when death occurred in an acute hospital, 41.5 percent when it occurred in another inpatient setting such as a nursing home). Although it is not shown in table 8.4, most PCPs who were dissatisfied with where the patient died would have preferred that the death had occurred at home (59 percent of those who were dissatisfied) or in an inpatient hospice setting (28 percent of those who were dissatisfied). This pattern of relationships strongly suggests that family members value the notion of patients' dying at home, a fact that becomes most family-evident when members have been disappointed.

When the PCP was asked whether he or she felt that the patient remained at home as long as he or she wanted, 72.4 percent of all responses were negative (see table 8.5). For patients who died at home, 96.5 percent of the PCP respondents felt that the patients were at home as much as they had wanted. On the other hand, for patients who died in an inpatient setting, only one-half of the PCPs reported that patients spent as many of their final days at home as they had wanted. This difference suggests that, even retrospectively, family members view the patients' being at home as valued—something they feel the patient would have wanted, and possibly something that they feel guilty about not having actualized.

Satisfaction as a Function of Treatment Modality

We examined the prevalence of satisfaction with the site of death as measured by dissatisfaction with the site of death and whether the patient was home as

Table 8.4 PCP Satisfaction with the Patient's Site of Death by Actual Site of Death

	Actual Site of Death (Percentage)				
	Home (N = 602)	Inpatient Hospice (N = 328)	Acute Hospital (N = 442)	Other Inpatient Setting (N = 41)	Total (N = 1,413)
PCP Preferred Different Site of Death					
No	93.9	88.7	75.6	58.5	85.9
Yes	6.1	11.3	24.4	41.5	14.1

Table 8.5   PCP Report of Whether the Patient was Able to Stay at Home as Long as Wanted by Actual Site of Death

	Actual Site of Death (Percentage)				
	Home (N = 600)	Inpatient Hospice (N = 319)	Acute Hospital (N = 423)	Other Inpatient Setting (N = 42)	Total (N = 1,384)
Patient Able to Stay Home as Long as Wanted					
Yes	96.5	55.5	53.9	42.9	72.4
No	3.5	44.5	46.1	57.1	27.6

long as desired. To adjust for differences in the three samples, comparative analyses were derived from logistic regression procedures in which the two dependent variables were statistically adjusted for independent variables found to be related to the dependent measure and/or that were differentially distributed across the three samples. The resulting estimates in table 8.6 reveal what the average demonstration hospice PCP response would have been in the three settings.

PCPs involved in either the home-based or hospital-based system were significantly less likely to have preferred a different site of death than was the case for PCPs of nonhospice patients. This difference is not attributable to where patients actually died—only 27 percent of HB patients died at home, yet 88 percent of PCPs in HB systems were satisfied. Another way to consider this aspect of satisfaction is that despite the fact that HC patients were nearly twice as likely to die at home, there was no significant difference between the groups in the proportion of PCPs reported to be dissatisfied with where the patient died.

These samples also differed with respect to the proportion of PCPs reporting that the patient had been home as long as had been desired. As can be seen, the answer was yes for 82 percent of the HC respondents, but only 69 percent and 56 percent for HB and nonhospice respondents, respectively. All three paired comparisons are statistically significantly different. Clearly, PCPs are express-

Table 8.6   Adjusted Estimate of Proportion of PCPs Who Preferred a Different Site of Death and Proportion of PCPs Reporting Patient Was Home as Long as Desired by Sample

	Study Sample (Percentage)		
	Home-Care Hospice	Hospital-Based Hospice	Conventional Care
PCP Preferred Different Site of Death			
No	91	88	74
Yes	9	12	26
PCP Reports Patient Home as Long as Wanted			
Yes	82	6	56
No	18	31	44

Table 8.7   Satisfaction with Site of Death for Patients in Three Sample Groups Based upon Where the Patient Died

	Study Sample (Percentage)		
	Home-Care Hospice	Hospital-Based Hospice	Conventional Care
Patient Died at Home	63	27	13
Of these cases, PCPs satisfied with Pt's site of death	94	93	94
Patient Died in Inpatient Setting	37	73	87
Of these cases, PCPs satisfied with Pt's site of death	77	86	73

ing a preference for patients' being at home longer than they are. The home-care hospice model meets that desire more than the HB model and even more so than the nonhospice approach. Comparing the two measures, it is clear that only a small minority of PCPs were unhappy about where the patient died, but a larger minority would have liked the patient to be at home longer. This suggests that relative to their own and their families' preferences, patients in hospital-based hospice and nonhospice systems are hospitalized too early.

Table 8.7 attempts to synthesize these interrelationships. As can be seen, over 90 percent of PCPs whose patients died at home were satisfied with where the patient died, regardless of treatment setting or sample. A substantially smaller percentage of those PCPs with patients dying in an inpatient setting reported that they were satisfied, except for those patients and PCPs served by HB hospices where the satisfaction differential due to site of death is only seven percentage points. Thus, many of our findings regarding satisfaction with site of death are rooted in the proportion of patients actually dying at home.

Summary of Findings

The HC type of hospice has shown the more obvious ability to meet the expressed desires of patients and families for a home-oriented type of care. Clearly, the values of PCPs in the three care systems are very similar. It is the values of the HC patients/PCPs that are most likely to be met by virtue of the HC emphasis upon home-based care.

There are differences in the probability of patients dying at home as a function of the type of treatment setting to which they were exposed. These differences occur even controlling for where the patient was when initially entered in the study as well as for other factors that differentiate the samples. If served by an agency with beds, terminal cancer patients are more likely to die there. This relationship is particularly striking in the hospice group. Among HB hospices there is considerable variability with respect to the control hospice staff have over the use of the inpatient beds. While there was variability among the HB hospices with respect to the proportion of patients staying at home, in no case did the proportion of HB deaths at home approach that of any of the HC hospices.

Like all measures of satisfaction, satisfaction with site of death is generally high, but significantly lower among CC PCPs. Patients served in HC settings were more likely to have been at home as long as they had wanted—another measure of satisfaction—than was the case for either HB or CC patients. Our analyses of satisfaction suggest that there was less congruence between actuality and reported desire among HB and CC patients than among HC patients.

At least three important questions about satisfaction with site of death were neither addressed nor answered by this study. First, the PCPs were not asked to specify the precise sources of their satisfaction or dissatisfaction, that is, what was it about a death at home that was valued highly, and what was it about a death in an acute hospital or other institution that was valued negatively? Future research on this topic could provide information useful in improving satisfaction with terminal care in conventional as well as hospice settings.

Second, the judgments of satisfaction or dissatisfaction made by PCPs soon after the patients' deaths cannot be assumed to remain stable over time. It is well known that cognitive and affective orientations often shift in the months following initial bereavement reactions (see chapter 9).

Finally, this study did not distinguish between attitudes toward *dying* versus *living* in hospital and institutional settings. The conclusion that satisfaction was less frequent among PCPs whose family members died away from home does not necessarily represent an orientation toward home death as a general social value. A loss in perceived social value, for example, has often been associated with placement in a long-term-care facility. The dissatisfaction effect, then, might be based in part upon the fact that the patient had been living and receiving care away from home, and not entirely upon the additional fact that death occurred away from home.

Nevertheless, the available findings do suggest that HB hospices may be doing something different from CC settings. Hospital-based PCPs are more likely to be satisfied with where the patients died and are more likely to feel that patients remained at home as long as they wanted than was the case for CC PCPs. In addition, the HB settings differed in many respects from the traditional oncology ward in an acute hospital. Many, although not all, participating HB settings went to great effort to create a "homelike" environment as was originally espoused by the English originators of the hospice ideal. The homelike environment created by HB staff may have resulted in reducing the impact on patients of leaving their homes to spend their last days in an institutional setting. Since chapter 4 revealed that HB patients spend nearly as much time in an inpatient setting as do CC patients, an HB inpatient setting may provide an alternate form of treatment, one that approximates the desires of the PCP more than conventional care, allowing them to alter their perspective on the relative values of remaining at home.

9

The First Months of Bereavement

SYLVIA SHERWOOD,
ROBERT KASTENBAUM,
JOHN N. MORRIS,
AND SUSAN M. WRIGHT

The philosophy of hospice care encompasses a broad spectrum of time, place, and person. There is concern for the entire family unit as well as for the dying person. Comfort is to be provided whether the patient is at home or in a hospital bed. Furthermore, the hospice mission does not end abruptly at the moment of death. Hospice care also has the objective of alleviating the survivors' distress. Bereavement-related experiences and outcomes are not only of intrinsic interest, then, but comprise part of the basic evaluation agenda as well. The National Hospice Study had the opportunity to examine some of the most significant correlates of bereavement within the first three to four months following death. Before describing the methods and major findings it will be useful to identify a set of key questions and concerns.

Bereavement: Key Terms and Concepts

The clinical and research literature on bereavement has grown rapidly in recent decades. *The Anatomy of Bereavement* (Raphael 1983), for example, draws upon approximately four hundred references and represents only a judicious selection of the available material. Assumptions about bereavement have also grown rapidly, often running ahead of the data base. Attention will be limited here to adult bereavement and to those facets that are most germane to the evaluation of hospice care.

Bereavement, grief, mourning, anticipatory grief, pathological grief, stressful life event, and *secondary morbidity* are terms frequently encountered in the literature. The concept of a *good* or *appropriate* death is also important here. Each of these terms will be examined briefly to establish a clear vocabulary for the following analyses and discussions.

Bereavement refers to the objective status of the survivor. We are bereaved when a person close to us has died. The concept of bereavement is most useful when it is restricted to the objective fact of survivorship (Kastenbaum 1986). The fact that a woman has the status of a wife, for example, does not in itself convey any reliable information about the satisfactions, stresses, and meanings associated with this role in her life. Similarly, to learn that this wife has become a widow is a significant piece of information but does not justify assumptions about the experience, meaning, and consequences of this transition. The simple fact of bereavement can usually be established by objective methods. The *impact* of bereavement upon the individual, however, can only be determined through careful and systematic follow-up. The tendency of some writers to equate the status of being bereaved with any particular set of cognitions, emotional states, or social and physical consequences begs the questions that must be asked anew in every instance.

Grief is a *response* to the fact of bereavement. It is not the only possible response (a survivor may also feel relief, for example, that a long period of suffering has ended for the deceased), but it is a response that arouses particular concern because of the emotional pain involved and other possible negative consequences. Whether grief is described by clinicians, behavioral scientists, or by the suffering individuals themselves, it emerges as a pervasive disturbance of adaptive functioning. A classic description by Lindemann (1944) portrays many of the somatic features seen in acute grief:

> . . . sensations of somatic distress occurring in waves lasting from 20 minutes to an hour at a time, a feeling of tightness in the throat, choking with shortness of breath, need for sighing, an empty feeling in the abdomen, lack of muscular power, and an intensive subjective distress described as tension or pain. (Lindemann 1944, 145)

The total state of grief is also likely to involve cognitive components such as difficulties with memory and concentration. Physical functions such as sleep and appetite are often affected, and the sufferer may have problems in carrying out ordinary responsibilities at home and work. Anxiety and depression are so characteristic a part of the reaction that some have defined grief as essentially just another name for a depressed anxiety that is experienced after the loss of an important person (e.g., Switzer 1970). Leaving aside for the moment the various specific theories that have been offered on this subject, grief presents itself as a general state of dysphoria with manifestations and correlates in every realm of functioning. Unlike the status of bereavement, the response known as grief can be precipitated by many causes other than the death of a loved one (loss of a relationship for reasons other than death, failure of a major career goal, and so on).

Mourning is the culturally patterned expression of response to the death of a person significant to the survivor. Such practices as the wearing of black arm bands or "widow's weeds," once more prevalent in our society, served as clear and instant signals of bereavement status. The specific forms taken by mourning are based upon varied cultural attitudes and traditions and are also subject to change over time. Some social scientists have proposed that new "rules" are needed to help people understand what is expected of them in situations (such as funerals) that once were united by consensual understanding (Calhoun and Selby 1985). Mourning practices are not only complex and sometimes ambiguous but also have varying relationships to the individual's actual experience and intent. A survivor who is relatively unperturbed by a particular death may engage in mourning behavior to "pay respects" and avoid social disapproval, while another bereaved person may have a devastating grief reaction but not be in a situation in which mourning seems appropriate. (In our mobile society, for example, it is not unusual for people to find themselves among "strangers" whom they do not want to burden with personal sorrows.)

The next terms have become important for their association with particular research and intervention approaches. It is not always easy to distinguish the factual core of each concept from its overlay of assumptions.

Anticipatory grief was introduced by Lindemann in 1944. The concept of anticipatory grief has become of increasing interest in recent years. Rando (1986) defines anticipatory grief as a broad phenomenon "stimulated and begun in part in response to the awareness of the impending loss of a loved one and the recognition of associated losses in the past, present, and future" (Rando 1986, 24). In reviewing current knowledge and usages, Rando emphasizes that anticipatory grief "takes time to unfold and develop. It is a process, not an all-or-nothing thing" (25). As will be seen below, anticipatory grief has come to be regarded as a positive phenomenon in the sense that it enables a person to work through some of the emotional distress and social discontinuities ahead of time and thereby reduce somewhat the impact of the death when it does occur. The unadorned basic concept, however, is simply that grief does not necessarily wait until the final loss is experienced, and that identifying and understanding this anticipatory process can be valuable to all persons involved.

Pathological grief is a term important for its interaction with its assumed opposite, *normal* grief. Attempts have been made for many years to distinguish between a form of grief that requires special attention to protect the individual from psychosocial or physical catastrophe, and a sequence of sorrow and distress that will run its course without serious long-term consequences. Examining the procession of claims and assertions over the past half century, one detects the gradual erosion of categorical thinking. Once it was assumed that a sharp differentiation could be made between pathological and normal forms of grief. Greater awareness of cultural and individual differences, however, and the limited utility of ostensibly differentiating criteria have generated a more cautious attitudinal climate. There is little doubt that some grief reactions are both devastating and dangerous, and little doubt that potentially severe reactions should be identified as soon as possible. Nevertheless, knowledgeable clinicians and researchers now show less inclination to base their approaches upon categorical distinctions between "pathological" and "normal" types of reaction.

Stressful life event. Bereavement can be interpreted as but one type of stressful life event. Although the nature of bereavement and the pattern of response may be distinctive in many ways, it is also plausible that some characteristics are shared with the larger set of phenomena known as stressful life events. The death of a loved one was recognized as among the most stressful life events by Holmes and Rahe (1967) when they started their pioneering work in this area. Because extensive research has now been done on a variety of stressful life events, studies of bereavement can be included within this larger domain. One of the major questions in the NHS exploration of the early bereavement period derives from previous research into stressful life events. Although the findings are not always consistent, the weight of the evidence from the literature tends to support the hypothesis that bereavement places at least some individuals at greater risk for adverse mental and physical health outcomes (e.g., Elliot and Eisdorfer 1982; Klerman and Izen 1977; Vachon 1976). What influence, if any, does hospice care in its two major organizational forms have upon bereavement as a stressful life event?

Secondary morbidity. The illness and disability of the terminally ill person comprise the primary morbidity of concern in the NHS. Secondary morbidity refers to difficulties in the physical, cognitive, emotional, or social spheres of functioning that may be experienced by those closely involved with the terminally ill person. The concept of secondary morbidity can be extended to all family members, neighbors, colleagues, and professional and volunteer caregivers. Within the limits of the NHS, however, attention was focused on the well-being of the primary caregiver. Specific indices of secondary morbidity serve as operational measures of the stressful life experience associated both with providing care to a terminally ill family member and in coping with the subsequent bereavement.

Appropriate death. As the awareness of the death movement became more articulate in the United States (see chapter 1), there also developed an implicit concept of the "good" or "desirable" death. (Actually, the discussion usually centered on the quality of life during the terminal phase of life, rather than death per se, but common usage often blurs this distinction.) It was unacceptable that a person should die in pain and social isolation. There must be, then, some more positive ideal or model for "dying well," perhaps a modern counterpart to such historical versions as Jeremy Taylor's (1651/1977). This is not the place to describe and analyze the various conceptions that have surfaced in recent years. It is useful to take an instructive example, however. A psychiatrist with extensive clinical and research experience in terminal care offered the concept of an "appropriate death." By this term, Avery D. Weisman (1972) means the death a person would have chosen for himself or herself—were a choice really possible. This concept has the advantage of clarity without overspecificity, and of recognizing individual differences while still holding on to a general rule. Whether or not one endorses Weisman's concept, it is likely that *some* image of "the good death" or "dying well" influences the attitudes and actions of everybody involved with terminal care and its evaluation.

Assumptions and Questions

The specific bereavement-related questions explored by the NHS were selected with two major criteria in mind: (1) relevance to the study's basic mission, and (2) congruence with available clinical observations and research findings. Additionally, of course, it was considered important to limit the response burden as much as possible and to remain within the established constraints of time and money. Many rounds of vigorous discussion made it clear that no matter which hard choices were made, it would not be possible to study all the variables that could be important in understanding the relationship between hospice care and bereavement outcome. The following summary of basic assumptions and questions will explicate the approach finally taken. Some of the significant alternatives *not* taken in the present study because of operational constraints are discussed in chapter 13, along with other thoughts concerning a future research agenda.

A Broad Spectrum of Possible Outcomes Should Be Studied

The assumption that bereavement constitutes a stressful life event appeared well justified by the work of previous investigators. Studies within the stressful-life-event framework had already identified many aspects of the individual's total functioning that were vulnerable to the fact of bereavement and the response of grief. There was no firm basis, however, for selecting any one domain of functioning as either more significant than others or as providing a more appropriate test of hospice care. Sampling a broad spectrum of outcome measures appeared to be a more effective strategy both for evaluation and for adding to our general knowledge of bereavement effects.

A specific guiding principle was applied to the selection process: give priority to those measures that have been found to differentiate between a nonbereaved population and those who have suffered a loss by death within the past few months. Previous studies had found that various measures of emotional stress, depression, and anxiety did make this differentiation (e.g., Parkes 1965; Clayton and Darvish 1979). Additionally, physical symptoms of the "psychosomatic" type described by Lindemann (1944) also appeared to be more characteristic of those recently bereaved than of nonbereaved individuals. Loss of weight and weight fluctuations were found by Marris (1958), Maddison and Viola (1968), and Parkes and Brown (1972). Indigestion, dizziness, fainting, trembling, or twitching were found to be more common in recently bereaved than in nonbereaved populations by Maddison and Viola (1968), and Parkes and Brown (1972). Sleeplessness and palpitations were found by some of the previously cited investigators as well as Clayton et al. (1974) and Glick, Weiss, and Parkes (1974).

Disturbances had been found in the realm of interpersonal relationships by many previous investigators. Loneliness emerged as a particularly salient outcome in studies of recent widows and widowers by Ball (1976–77) and Carey (1979–80). The interpersonal domain appeared particularly important for the NHS since the hospice approach places a strong emphasis on maintaining social relationships.

Numerous measures have been employed to investigate risk for physical illness and poor health status. It is important to note that predictors of poor health status are themselves not limited to the physical domain. Increases in the utilization of health-care resources have proven to be especially relevant in examining the short-term effects of bereavement. Particular attention has been given to doctor visits and acute hospitalizations (e.g., Weiner et al. 1975, and several studies previously cited). The research literature also suggests that poor mental health prior to bereavement is also a major predictor of poor bereavement outcome (e.g., Clayton 1982; Bunch 1972; Theorell 1974; Andrews et al. 1978). Questions can also be raised about the interaction between emotional reactions during the "anticipatory grief" phase preceding death and bereavement outcome. Can poor emotional and physical health reactions in the early months of bereavement be predicted by dysphoric mood and low morale in the period immediately preceding death? Is the degree to which care of the patient was felt as a burden predictive of poor bereavement outcomes? Questions such as these have been suggested, but their answers not conclusively provided, by previous studies. It is possible, for example, that the anxiety and depression expressed prior to the death of a loved one actually constitutes a positive, if painful, phase of anticipatory grief. Similarly, it could also be hypothesized that the greater the felt burden of patient care, then the greater the relief when the struggle is ended, leading to a quicker adjustment to the loss.

Bereavement outcomes were conceptualized in terms of a number of domains, including emotional, social, and physical components. It was not assumed that these domains are functionally isolated from each other; rather, the relationships among all the events and processes were considered to be of great interest. The methodology applied to the challenge of examining bereavement outcomes (see below) would be intended, then, to sample these domains as adequately as possible within the project constraints and with particular emphasis on those changes most likely to occur within the first months following bereavement.

The Possible Effects of Differential Care Systems upon Bereavement
Outcomes Should Be Clearly Evaluated

This objective was intrinsic to the mission of NHS. It was not enough, however, to establish a set of outcome variables and analyze them by type of care system (home-based hospice, hospital-based hospice, and conventional care). It was also important to recognize the somewhat conflicting assumptions and expectations involved. A few of the most salient alternatives are summarized below.

1. *The hospice approach places a heavier burden on the primary care person (PCP)—therefore, a pattern indicative of greater stress will be found, as compared with the conventional-care system.* This excess burden and its predicted negative consequences should also be more evident within the home-based type of hospice organization as compared with the hospital-based (the conventional-care approach, requiring the least daily caregiving effort from the PCP, should also result in the lowest index of secondary morbidity and other negative bereavement outcomes).

2. *The hospice approach is more supportive of the relationship between patient and PCP, and more conducive to the emotional comfort of both— therefore, the bereavement outcome should be less negative for those enrolled in hospice programs.* The overall pattern should prove to be the obverse of the pattern suggested by the burden hypothesis. The conventional-care approach, with its greater emphasis on aggressive testing and treatment within the hospital setting, should produce the most disruption in the patient-PCP relationship, and so provide the least protection against negative bereavement oucomes, followed by the hospital-based hospice approach, with the home-based approach proving most effective in alleviating the PCP's distress after the patient's death.

3. *Most people adjust to the particular circumstances they face—therefore there will be no clear differential pattern of bereavement outcome related to type of care system.* This hypothesis does not seem to appear in either the hospice or bereavement literature. Nevertheless, it is possible that both advocates and critics of the hospice approach have underestimated the flexibility and personal resources of the "average" person. Some people have functioned well and achieved notably despite a variety of stresses and deprivations. It may be, then, that something about the individual's overall resiliency and coping ability could prove to be more influential than the particular advantages and disadvantages encountered within the three types of care systems studied here.

The three alternative hypotheses that have been described here could also have been worked for more specific predictions. It is not necessary to assume that each of the three processes emphasized by the various hypotheses would have equal influence upon all outcome domains. The hypothesis that centers around the burden generated by hospice care, for example, might show its main effects on reported sense of burden and physical fatigue. By contrast, the hypothesis based upon hospice care as support to the maintenance of interpersonal relationships might show its main effects on such variables as self-esteem and social interaction. Believing, however, that it would be premature to formulate highly specific hypotheses on the basis of the information available, it was decided to stay alert for possible differential outcomes but otherwise to wait for the data to speak for themselves.

Each Intervention Represents a Complex and Time-Sensitive Configuration, Not a Monolithic Independent Variable

Just as the bereavement outcome must be studied with respect to a spectrum of specific variables, so one must be aware that each of the three care systems comprises a complex set of operations, events, and processes. This means, at the very least, that we should not succumb to the temptation to regard each intervention as a simple "independent variable." Each modality of care—home-based hospice, hospital-based hospice, and conventional care—has its distinctive configuration of services and somewhat distinctive temporal patterns as well. Even assuming that clear differential effects are found on some outcome measures among the three care systems, this finding would not automatically establish which factors were the most decisive.

Consider, for example, one of the questions already examined in an earlier section of this book (chapter 8). Did the type of care provided have a differential effect on the probability of patients dying at home? The findings indicate that such an effect did occur. The probability of dying at home was a function of the type of treatment setting. Patients served by home-based hospices did in fact have a higher probability of dying at home than those served by agencies that operated their own inpatient facilities. This, of course, is a finding that could not have been known at the time the study was planned. With the results now available, though, it would be logical to look for the specific influence of site of death upon bereavement outcome measures. In other words, perhaps it was this fact and this fact only that made the difference in the nature of the bereavement response among PCPs—assuming, that is, that any such differences were actually to be found. This is but one simplified version of a process that would need to be repeated for every variable and every combination of variables that comprise the distinctive configuration of all three approaches to terminal care. There was not even any compelling reason to assume that the same variables would be of equal importance across the three types of care systems. How well pain was controlled, for example, might be the key variable that mediates bereavement outcomes for one care system, while for another care system the key might be the frequency of contacts with health-care personnel.

It was frustrating—but realistic—to acknowledge that the NHS would not be in a position to examine the independent and combinatory influence of all the intervention variables on all the outcome measures. A study designed with this as the sole purpose would have been a rather different one than the study actually undertaken in response to a larger set of questions linked to time-sensitive policy decisions. The NHS effort would have to be sensitive to the complexity of the different care systems participating in the demonstration program, but could not hope to answer fully all the questions that might be raised about the *specific* relationships between a given dimension of hospice or conventional-care intervention and a given dimension of bereavement outcome.

Early Bereavement Provides an Incomplete but Significant View of the Individual's Response to Loss

There was once a strong tendency to believe that people suffer the effects of a significant loss for about a year and then "get over it." Indices of grief and disorganization that endured beyond that supposedly normative allotment were considered to be indicative of either "pathology" or "self-indulgent weakness," depending upon one's frame of reference. However, as indicated earlier in this chapter, those familiar with the grief process now are less likely to impose arbitrary points for either the onset or the cessation of the grief response. Data from various sources suggest the existence of important individual differences (e.g., Sanders 1977) and the tendency for grief to be rekindled in brief but intense waves even when the death has receded many years into the past (e.g., Rosenblatt 1983).

This revised orientation toward grief and the life course seems to represent a more mature and realistic outlook. It is consistent with the observations of Erik Erikson (1982) and other writers who see the human condition as always vulnerable to threat and loss, but always demonstrating some capacity to interpret and cope with the sorrows and conflicts to which flesh is heir. In the ideal research situation, one would learn much about the individual's way of life and mode of coping with adversity prior to a significant death experience and then attempt to trace the effects of this experience throughout the entire remaining course of life. It is obvious that in this as well as in other areas, the NHS could provide not the ideal study but the study that could be done effectively and productively within the limits imposed.

Nevertheless, if one had to select a limited time span within which to examine bereavement-related outcomes, it is likely that most researchers would make the choice that was ours without choice: the several months immediately following death of the loved one. A number of studies indicate that the development of grief reactions tends to be fairly rapid (e.g., Engel 1961; Clayton et al. 1974). The highest levels of grief were found by Klerman and Izen (1977) to occur within the first four months of bereavement. Those survivors who show the most disturbed pattern over an extended period of time are most often those with the greatest level of disturbance soon after bereavement (Parkes and Brown 1972; Bornstein et al. 1973; Vachon et al. 1982).

With the exception of mortality, it can be anticipated that bereavement outcomes of exceptional severity, if they did occur, would have been likely to show themselves during the period covered by the NHS analysis. Mortality, even among the bereaved, is an infrequent event over a period of a year, and the research literature suggests that the period of peak risk occurs in the second six months following bereavement. Furthermore, men forty-five and under whose wife or mother has died appear to be the group at greatest risk (Klerman and Izen 1977). In the NHS samples, only a very small percent (2 percent or less in each of the three samples) are widowers of forty-five or younger. Even when all men forty-five or under who lost a mother are combined with the young widower group, only some 4 percent are in this category (3 percent in the HC, and 4 percent each in the HB and CC groups). Given the small numbers who can be expected to die among these subgroups within a three- or four-month period, it is not very meaningful to analyze for differential effects. Mortality, therefore, was not included as one of the PCP outcome variables in the analysis of the differential impact of the three types of terminal care systems.

Method

The analytic procedures for determining the impact of hospices on the first months of bereavement of principal care persons of deceased hospice patients were similar to those used in evaluating the impact of hospices on patient quality of life described in chapter 7.

Guiding Questions

The general consideration of assumptions and problems led to the formulation of a more specific set of guiding questions. The major question for the NHS was clearly: *Are there differences in the impact of hospital-based hospice programs (HB), home-based hospice programs (HC), and conventional care (CC) on mental, social, and physical-health bereavement outcomes for the principal care persons (PCPs) of terminally ill cancer patients?*

A more specific set of questions was then derived: *What is the impact of hospital-based as compared with home-based hospices and conventional care on:*

1. the *emotional stress* experienced by the PCP during the months immediately following bereavement?
2. the *social reengagement* of the PCP during the bereavement period?
3. the *number of doctor visits* made by the PCP during the bereavement period?
4. the *anxiety/depression* felt by the PCP *prior* to the death of the patient?

5. the extent to which helping in the care of the patient prior to death is *perceived as a burden* by the PCP?
6. the PCP's *satisfaction with the health and service support care* both prior to and following the patient's death?
7. the extent of *bereavement counseling* received by the PCP?
8. the PCP's *dissatisfaction with bereavement counseling?*

Additional questions were also formulated and tested to explore certain risk factors for negative bereavement outcomes across the three groups. These analyses are reported later in the present chapter.

Sample

The analyses reported in this chapter utilize self-report data from PCPs participating in the follow-up sample (see chapter 2). The study group includes all PCPs in the follow-up sample who completed a bereavement interview. Excluded in this analysis are PCPs for patients who did not die within the time frame of the NHS. Basic characteristics of PCPs in all three groups are given in table 9.1.

Although the terminally ill cancer patients were almost equally divided among males and females, most of the PCPs (72 percent) were female. The mean age of a PCP was fifty-eight years. About half were married to the patient, and only about 5 percent were classified as nonrelatives. Most PCPs (more than 90 percent) were married. As might be expected given their relationship, PCPs and patients presented similar profiles in terms of race and religion (demographic information given in chapter 2). Fewer than 10 percent of the PCPs were nonwhite. The HC sample was about 55 percent Protestant and 28 percent Catholic, while the other two samples were each in the 40 percent range for both Protestants and Catholics. The HC sample had a higher percent of Jewish PCPs (about 10 percent) than did the other samples (5 percent HB and 3 percent CC).

Because some demographic differences did exist among the three samples it was necessary to introduce a statistical procedure that would control for the imperfect intergroup match. Multiple linear regression procedures were employed to adjust for the differences. This procedure has been described in chapter 7. A thoroughly detailed account can be found in the technical report prepared by NHS for the Health Care Financing Administration (obtainable from the National Technical Information Service).

Sources of Data

Data focusing on PCPs and their life situations were collected at three points in time. The initial interview conducted with the PCP at study intake asked specific questions about the respondents' life situations. A follow-up interview

Table 9.1   Percentage Distributions by Samples of PCP Characteristics

	HC (N ≈ 780)	HB (N ≈ 580)	CC (N ≈ 270)
Demographics			
Age			
21–44	19.9	20.6	29.2
45–54	16.8	15.9	15.8
55–64	21.0	22.8	29.5
65–74	30.1	29.4	17.8
75+	12.2	11.3	7.7
Female	71.0	72.7	73.2
Relationship to Patient			
Spouse	57.5	51.0	52.0
Child	26.1	31.8	26.2
Other Relative	11.1	13.7	17.1
Nonrelative	5.3	3.5	4.7
Single	7.1	9.4	9.4
Nonwhite	8.1	5.3	9.2
Completed High School	76.9	74.5	73.3
Employed at Intake	29.1	39.0	40.5
Household Income			
Less than 5K	11.9	12.4	14.4
$5–10K	30.2	27.3	25.8
$10–20K	30.5	33.2	33.0
$20–30K	15.4	15.1	12.1
$30–50K	8.4	9.5	11.0
$50K+	3.6	2.5	3.8
Household Income Change in Last Year			
Decrease	16.0	15.7	14.7
No Change	60.4	66.4	62.6
Increase	23.6	17.9	22.7
Religion			
Protestant	54.7	40.5	41.9
Catholic	28.2	42.0	47.7
Jewish	9.5	5.3	2.7
Other	7.6	12.2	7.7
Religion Very Important	58.2	62.2	61.4
Social Supports			
Rates Family and Friends as Helpful and Supportive	84.2	85.2	84.5
Family Tension in Week of Intake	39.3	38.3	38.9
Physical Health			
Felt Well in Week of Intake	80.4	82.6	80.8
Health Condition Limits Helping Pt	40.7	34.1	30.7
Psychological Characteristics			
Difficulty Sleeping in Week of Intake	60.5	53.4	57.5
Satisfied with Ability to Meet Pt's Needs in Week of Intake	83.1	87.9	79.6
Medication for Nerves or Depression in Week of Intake	19.2	15.6	16.3

Table 9.1   *(cont.)*

	HC (N ≈ 780)	HB (N ≈ 580)	CC (N ≈ 270)
Multiple Stressors			
One or More Other Stresses	33.4	24.5	20.5
Length of Illness			
Less than one year	45.1	46.9	43.1
One to two years	15.7	17.6	18.7
Two to three years	10.6	8.3	11.4
More than three years	28.6	27.1	26.8

focusing on PCP concerns and life situation was conducted about three weeks later. The final data collection point was the bereavement interview, which took place, on the average, about three and a half months after the patient's death. Each interview had to be somewhat limited to prevent overburdening the PCP. The initial interview (including information about the patient as well as the PCP) took about twenty-five minutes, the follow-up interview about fifteen minutes, and about twenty-five minutes for the bereavement interview.

Bereavement outcome measures were based on PCP self-report data from the final interview. Outcomes prior to bereavement (anxiety/depression and felt burden of care) were based on the second interview. Data from the first interview provided descriptive characteristics of both the patient and the PCP that, along with patient intake record data and information gathered directly from the patients, were used as control variables in the analyses of hospice impact on PCP bereavement outcomes. Data from the first PCP interview and the patient intake record served as control variables in the analyses of prebereavement outcomes.

Dependent (Outcome) Measures

Despite the limitations imposed by time constraints and the need to minimize PCPs' response burden, the total set of measures was quite extensive: fifty-five separate items ultimately entered one or more of the regression analyses for the array of dependent outcome variables under investigation. These variables can be grouped as follows: (1) the PCP's emotional state at study intake (e.g., anxiety/depression, felt burden of care); (2) general health status of PCP at study intake; (3) family supports; (4) patient variables, such as length of illness, condition prior to death, and so on; (5) satisfaction with care provided to the patient at the point of intake into the study; and (6) demographics and other descriptors.

Table 9.2 lists each item, the scoring system (range of values), and the percentage of each of the three PCP study groups (HB, HC, CC) that had a selected score on the item.

Table 9.2 Independent Variables Entering Regression Equations (and Logit Analysis for DSCOU)

Variable	Category Range		Selected Category	% in Selected Categories		
				CC	HB	HC
Sex of PCP	1 Female	2 Male	Female	73.2	72.7	71.0
PCP is Catholic	1 No	2 Yes	Yes	47.7	42.0	28.2
PCP Education	1 0–8	5 16–24	High School Grad.	73.3	74.5	76.8
PCP is a Working Woman	0 No	1 Yes	Yes	25.5	23.3	16.6
PCP, under 46, Female, Not Working	0 No	1 Yes	Yes	13.7	11.7	7.0
Religiosity of PCP	1 Not Import.	4 Very Import.	Very Important	61.4	62.2	58.2
PCP Employment	1 No	2 Yes	Yes	40.5	39.0	29.9
Patient's Overall Quality of Life	0 Lowest	14 Highest	6 or Less	39.7	46.6	53.7
Patient's Functional Assessment	1 Best	4 Worst	Worst	41.4	27.2	22.2
HRCA Quality of Life—1st Assessment (Patient)	0 Worst	10 Best	8–10	5.3	4.2	4.7
HRCA Quality of Life Closest to Death (Patient)*	0 Worst	10 Best	6 or Less	93.8	94.0	94.9
Patient's Initial Karnofsky	1 Worst	5 Best	Less than 5	94.5	85.2	83.0
PCP over 64 Years/Illness More than 1 Year	0 No	1 Yes	Yes	16.6	21.5	23.9
Days from Initial Interview to Death	0 Same Day	329 329 Days	Less than 15 Days	29.0	30.1	24.6
PCP—Felt Well	1 Yes	2 No	Yes	80.8	82.6	80.4
PCP—Plenty of Energy	1 Yes	2 No	Yes	61.0	64.2	59.6
PCP—Change in Appetite	1 Yes	2 No	No	66.3	65.4	60.4
PCP—Difficulty Sleeping	1 Yes	2 No	Yes	57.5	53.4	60.5
PCP—Headaches	1 Yes	2 No	Yes	29.6	28.5	29.7
PCP—Medication for Nerves	1 Yes	2 No	Yes	16.3	15.6	19.2
PCP—Increased Family Intimacy	1 Yes	2 No	Yes	59.5	63.1	69.2
Health Conditions Limit PCP	0 No	1 Yes	No	69.3	65.9	59.3
PCP—Cold Sweats	1 Yes	2 No	No	92.2	94.6	87.5

160

Variable						
PCP—Experienced Family Tension	1 Yes	2 No	Yes	38.9	38.3	39.3
Patient is Receiving Disability Insurance	1 Yes	2 No	Yes	22.2	9.9	14.0
% Outpatient Paid by Family Last 6 Months	1 None	4 Most	None	60.7	44.9	42.7
Blue Cross/Blue Shield	0 No	1 Yes	Yes	24.5	27.5	21.4
PCP's Household Income	1 <5K	6 50K+	10K–20K	33.0	33.3	30.5
Anxiety/Depression	0 Least	5 Most	Most	14.5	6.7	7.7
Feelings of Burden	0 Least	6 Most	Most	8.0	10.0	14.0
PCP Reduced Work Hours Because of Patient	0 No Change	1 Change	Change	27.3	27.5	28.3
PCP Reduced Response to Important Needs	0 Not at All	2 A Lot	Not at All	51.0	44.6	36.6
PCP has Other Life Crises	0 Least	2 Most	Least	79.5	75.5	66.5
PCP Life Complicated by Other Crises	1 Not at All	3 A Lot	A Lot	16.0	15.4	23.8
PCP Mentions Patient is Dying	1 Mentioned	2 Not Mentioned	Mentioned	61.6	72.3	72.8
Nonhospice Doctor/Nurses Involved in Care Decisions	1 Yes	2 No	No	22.0	36.9	28.1
PCP Instrumental Support	0 Hours	6 225–336 Hours	0 Hours	14.6	10.6	1.8
Past Week Time Patient Chatted with Housemates	1 None	4 Considerable	None	17.3	16.7	9.5
# Family/Friends Patient Can Rely On	1	7 10+	10+	23.3	13.8	14.4
Family/Friends Helpful, Supportive	1 Agree	2 Disagree	Agree	84.5	85.2	84.2
# Patient's Living Children	0 0	5 5–15	0	17.6	18.1	14.7
Doctor Tells Patient All	0 Disagree	1 Agree	Agree	77.3	76.8	73.0
Doctor Lets Patient Discuss Thoughts	0 Disagree	1 Agree	Agree	86.1	83.7	81.8
Family Involved in Treatment Decisions	1 Mentioned	2 Not Mentioned	Not Mentioned	39.5	29.7	35.9
PCP Satisfied with Patient's Counseling	0 Disagree	1 Agree	Agree	61.7	82.0	75.6

(contd.)

Table 9.2 Independent Variables Entering Regression Equations (and Logit Analysis for DSCOU) (*contd.*)

Variable	Category Range		Selected Category	% in Selected Categories		
				CC	HB	HC
PCP Satisfied with Medical Care of Patient	0 Disagree	1 Agree	Agree	86.1	91.2	86.7
PCP Satisfied with Ability to Meet Patient's Needs	1 Yes	2 No	Yes	79.6	87.9	83.1
Patient has Short Breath	0 No	1 Yes	Yes	57.8	51.9	56.6
Colon Cancer	0 No	1 Yes	No	86.7	83.0	86.8
Aggressive Cancer Care	1 Aggressive	2 Other	Aggressive	35.0	13.1	20.0
Last 6 Months Doctor Recommended Operation	0 No	1 Yes	Yes	50.6	43.8	45.1
Days in Institution, Month of Intake	0 No Days	1 One+	No Days	98.9	86.0	98.6
Patient Lives with PCP	1 Yes	2 No	Yes	70.5	70.2	86.4
PCP Married to Someone Not Patient	0 No	1 Yes	No	74.2	72.7	75.6
PCP is Spouse of Patient	1 Yes	2 No	Yes	52.0	57.0	57.4

Note: Except for the independent variable identified with an asterisk, all variables are baseline measures (i.e., gathered at study intake).

Within the interview time restraints of this study it was not possible to develop separate scales for each of the variables within a domain of outcome variables identified in the literature. However, a series of key scales (alpha reliabilities of 0.5 or higher) were constructed and are sensitive to the type of outcomes most likely to appear in the first months of bereavement. The most extensive and important of these is the emotional stress scale, which itself builds upon several other scales: unsettled/anxious, overwhelmed/depressed, tension/anger, somatic (bodily) symptoms, and change in appetite/weight. Additionally, it was possible to use a number of single items from the PCP bereavement interview to examine some of these areas.

All but two of these analyses involved constructed scales. Because the presence of emotional problems was considered the most crucial outcome on which hospice care might have a positive impact, the analysis of differential effect of HB, HC, and CC on PCPs' emotional stress will be presented first, followed by examination of differential effect on anxiety/depression during the prebereavement period. Findings concerning the two remaining key bereavement domains will then be presented. The last set of analyses pertain to the remaining prebereavement outcomes and the three intervening bereavement outcomes. Listed in the order of presentation, then, the dependent measures for analyses are:

- emotional stress.
- anxiety/depression (prebereavement).
- social reengagement.
- number of physician visits.
- feelings of burden (prebereavement).
- extent of bereavement counseling scale.
- dissatisfaction with bereavement counseling.
- satisfaction with patient care (measured prior to and after the patient's death).

Operational definitions and score distributions for each of the selected dependent variables are presented in detail in the appropriate sections below.

Findings

Major findings of the impact analysis are summarized to begin this section. Detailed results are then presented in the same sequence for each research question: the dependent variable and its distribution of scores is described, followed by a graphic illustration of the overall impact assessment. (Specific regression equations for each outcome variable can be found in the NHS technical report obtainable from the National Technical Information Service.)

Major Results

Key findings from the impact analysis on eight dependent variables (table 9.3) can be summarized as follows:

1. Emotional-stress scores of PCPs in the hospital-based hospice group did not differ from those in the conventional-care sample when interviewed about three and a half months after the patients' death. However, a significant difference was found between PCPs in the two hospice groups. The PCPs of hospital-based patients were less emotionally distressed than were the PCPs of home-care patients.

2. No differences in anxiety/depression outcome were found in PCPs as a function of type of terminal care provided (HB, HC, CC).

3. Social reengagement after the death of the patient was significantly higher for the PCPs of home-care hospice as compared with those of hospital-based hospice patients.

4. The number of PCP doctor visits from the time of the patient's death to the bereavement interview did not differ significantly across the three samples.

5. No differences were found between the PCPs of CC patients and either hospice sample in the feelings of burden resulting from patient care while the patient was still living. There was, however, a significant difference between the two hospice samples, with the PCPs of hospital-based patients having lower feelings of burden than the PCPs of home-care patients.

6. Significantly more bereavement counseling was received by PCPs of home-care hospice patients than by PCPs in the other two groups.

Table 9.3   Summary of Adjusted Means for PCP of Average Hospice Patient on Specified Dependent Variables

	Adjusted Means			z Score Comparisons		
	HC	HB	CC	CC vs. HB	CC vs. HC	HB vs. HC
Emotional Stress	5.06	4.49	4.82	1.45	1.07	3.41
Anxiety/Depression	2.96	2.98	3.01	0.27	0.44	0.20
Social Reengagement	1.45	1.29	1.41	1.14	0.41	2.08
Number of Doctor Visits	1.35	1.25	0.95	0.85	1.24	0.35
Feelings of Burden	3.32	2.91	3.13	1.19	1.09	3.49
Extent of Bereavement Counseling	1.63	1.36	1.36	0.01	2.49	3.06
Dissatisfaction with Bereavement Counseling	1.04	1.02	1.05	1.34	0.55	1.40
Satisfaction with Patient Care (assessed at follow-up)	4.39	4.54	4.38	1.59	0.15	2.30
Satisfaction with Patient Care (assessed at bereavement)	4.36	4.48	4.34	1.63	0.32	2.01

Table 9.4   Scoring of Emotional Stress

Bereavement Scales Subsumed		Scale Recodes		
Scale Title	Scale Range	No Problem	Some Problem	Greater Problem
Somatic (Bodily) symptoms	0–9	0	1, 2	3–9
Overwhelmed/depressed	0–13	0	1, 2	3–13
Changes in appetite/weight	0–2	0	1	2
Unsettled/anxious	0–6	0, 1	2, 3	4–6
Tension/anger	0–6	0	1	2–6

7. There were no significant differences across the three groups of PCPs in dissatisfaction-with-bereavement-counseling scores.

8. Satisfaction-with-patient-care scores revealed no significant differences between the hospice and conventional-care PCPs. However, for a period prior to the death of the patient, the PCPs of hospital-based hospice patients were significantly more satisfied with patient care than were the PCPs of home-care hospice patients.

More detailed descriptions and findings of the impact analyses now follow.

Emotional Distress

Two measures were utilized to examine the differential impact of HB, HC, and CC on the PCPs' emotional status. The key measure, emotional stress, focuses on bereavement outcomes. It is an eleven-point comprehensive scale, incorporating mood and psychosomatic variables. As indicated previously, the emotional-stress measure subsumes five highly correlated subscales. These subscales were developed by the HRCA research staff and are composed primarily of items from Sander's Grief Experience Inventory (Sanders 1977). The second measure is a five-item anxiety/depression scale that focuses on the prebereavement period.

The majority of PCPs in all three samples were not severely depressed, according to the distribution of scores on both measures of emotional distress (tables 9.4, 9.5, and 9.6). Fewer than 10 percent were in the worst response categories on each measure, while about 50 percent were in the middle or more positive categories.

The hospice alternatives did not appear to have a significant differential effect, either positive or negative, on the emotional outcomes of family members. There are no significant differences when conventional care is compared with hospice care regarding the emotional stress experienced by the principal care person during the first months of bereavement, although a difference was found between the two hospice groups. Figures 9.1 and 9.2 display the impact findings for each measure with statistical adjustments to control for intergroup differences at intake. Taken together, these findings suggest that there are no

Table 9.5   Percentage Distribution of Scores by Sample for
Adverse Emotional Response (by PCP) at Bereavement Interview

		CC	HB	HC
Most stress	10	9.1	4.7	6.3
	9	9.5	3.5	10.2
	8	8.6	7.1	11.0
	7	8.2	7.3	10.3
	6	10.9	11.8	9.8
	5	8.2	5.6	8.7
	4	9.5	10.8	11.9
	3	10.0	17.1	8.7
	2	10.0	12.5	8.9
	1	8.2	11.8	8.2
Least stress	0	7.7	7.8	6.0
Sample		Mean	Median	N
		5.06	5.06	220
		4.17	3.58	425
		5.17	5.22	620

Note: Scale developed by HRCA from other HRCA-developed
scales.

Table 9.6   Percentage Distribution of Scores by Sample for Anxiety/Depression (of PCP)
at Follow-up Interview Based on Five True/False Questions

		CC	HB	HC
Most Anxiety/Depression	5	15.5	10.0	8.9
	4	21.7	19.1	22.8
	3	19.9	20.1	20.9
	2	14.9	18.2	20.1
	1	18.6	19.1	18.4
Least Anxiety/Depression	0	9.3	13.5	8.9
Sample		Mean	Median	N
		2.73	2.86	161
		2.42	2.46	319
		2.57	2.63	473

*PCP reported in the past week:
  Feeling depressed
  Feeling fearful
  Not usually feeling happy
  Feeling under considerable pressure
  Feeling restless

differences in the proportion of PCPs experiencing higher levels of emotional
distress during the patients' last weeks of life. By the time of bereavement,
however, exposure to the hospital-based hospice program appears to have
resulted in a lessening of the proportion of PCPs in the higher categories of
emotional distress.

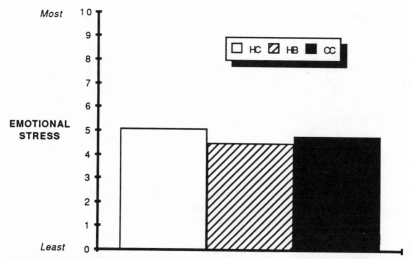

Figure 9.1   Mean Score on Adverse Emotional Stress for PCP of "Average" Hospice Patient at Bereavement

Social Reengagement

The home-care hospice alternative showed a significant superiority to hospital-based hospice programs in social reengagement during the first months of bereavement. The NHS data analysis procedure, adjusting for intake differences among the samples, finds that the PCP of an average hospice patient

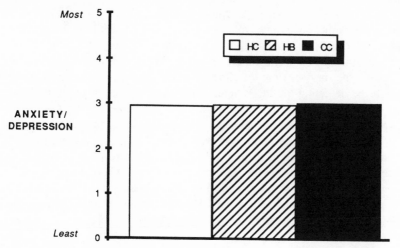

Figure 9.2   Mean Score on Anxiety/Depression for PCP of "Average" Hospice Patient at Follow-up Interview

Table 9.7   Percentage Distribution of Scores by Sample
for Social Reengagement (by PCP) after Death Based on Three Questions
about Social Activity

		CC	HB	HC
Most Increased Involvement	3	14.7	15.3	18.4
	2	26.7	24.6	31.4
	1	28.7	25.0	29.2
No Change or Decreased Involvement	0	29.8	35.1	21.0

Sample	Mean	Median	N
	1.26	1.20	258
	1.20	1.09	472
	1.47	1.49	701

Note: Scale developed by HRCA from Rand Corporation items.
PCP responded at bereavement interview to:
Has the amount of time you spend at leisure and recreational activities stayed
the same, decreased, or increased?
Has the amount of time you spend with relatives and friends stayed the same,
decreased, or increased?
What has happened to your ability to stay on top of family obligations?

would be more likely to have increased social involvement after the patient's
death if enrolled in a home-based hospice as compared with a hospital-based
hospice program. The largest component of this difference (see table 9.7)
appears to be the relatively smaller number of home-care PCPs whose social
involvement decreased after the death. The level of reengagement among HB
PCPs, however, was not greater than among those in conventional-care programs (fig. 9.3).

It is possible that the PCPs of home-care hospice patients disengaged the
most from other social involvements while they had such demanding responsibilities to perform on a daily basis. The patients' subsequent deaths may have
a powerful and complex impact on the PCPs' emotional state—but it also
liberates the survivor from the effort of protracted caregiving. The data, then,
might be depicting the PCPs' return to a more characteristic level of social
involvement. It is also possible that the PCPs of home-care hospice patients
experience a keener need for social reengagement once the patient has died.

It should be kept in mind, however, that the data all represent the PCPs'
perception of changes in social involvement. This perception is important in
itself, conveying as it does the family member's view of his or her life situation.
Nevertheless, there is still a need to examine changes in social involvement
from an objective standpoint as well. Direct measures of social reengagement
might or might not confirm the PCPs' perceptions.

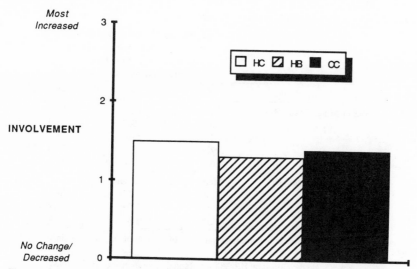

Figure 9.3   Mean Score on Social Reengagement for PCP of "Average" Hospice Patient at Bereavement

The Number of Physician Visits

The number of physician visits serves as an objective marker for the utilization of medical resources. (The possibility of charting specific diseases and impairments was considered in the NHS planning phase but was rejected because the frequency of occurrence was projected to be too low to permit meaningful analysis within the available time framework.) Increases in the number of physician visits during the first months of bereavement could serve as an indication of heightened susceptibility to illness. Table 9.8 provides the scoring and distribution of the three PCP groups on this variable. It can be seen that more than half of the PCPs had one or more consultations with a doctor in the relatively brief interval between the death of the patient and the bereavement interview. A little more than 10 percent in each group saw a doctor four or more times during this period of approximately three and a half months.

Figure 9.4 presents the impact findings, controlling for potential differences in the PCP groups at intake. PCPs in all three samples are comparable, with no significant differences emerging. In summary, there is no significant differential effect during this early bereavement period in the number of doctor visits made by the PCPs of conventional-care, hospital-based hospice, and home-care hospice patients.

Interesting to reflect upon but not investigated by NHS is the possibility that *avoidance* of medical attention can also be a response to stress. Relationships among health status, anxiety, and behavior have been shown to be highly

Table 9.8   Scoring of Number of Physician Visits

		Percentage Distribution of Scores by Sample for Number of Doctor Visits (by PCP) from Death to Bereavement Interview		
		CC	HB	HC
Four or More Visits	4	11.1	11.4	14.5
	3	6.1	6.2	9.9
	2	8.8	13.9	14.0
	1	27.6	25.1	22.5
No Visits	0	46.4	43.4	39.1
	Sample	Mean	Median	N
		1.08	0.63	261
		1.17	0.76	498
		1.38	0.99	724

Item: PCP report at bereavement interview of number of doctor visits since the death.

Note: Scale developed by HRCA from Rand Corporation and HRCA items.

complex, with paradoxical actions (or inaction) occurring often enough to require systematic investigation (e.g., Siegler and Costa 1985). One would also want to know more about the specific reasons for seeking doctor visits. It is possible, for example, that some PCPs neglected their own physical problems while focusing on those of the terminally ill patient and did not look after their own well-being until bereaved. It should not be assumed that all or even most doctor visits in the early months of bereavement were in response to conditions

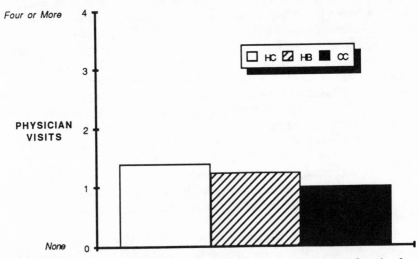

Figure 9.4   Mean Score on Number of Doctor Visits from Death to Bereavement Interview for PCP of "Average" Hospice Patient

caused or intensified by the stress of caring for a dying person.

Within the limits of the present study, however, it would appear that the number of doctor visits is a reasonable estimate of secondary morbidity, and that utilization of medical services did not occur at an alarmingly high level. As table 9.8 reveals, the preponderance of PCPs in all three samples had one doctor visit or none during the first three and a half months of bereavement. Taking into account the fact that many PCPs were older men and women who would be more susceptible to medical problems in any event, the utilization rate does not seem to be unusually high.

Feelings of Burden (Prebereavement)

It was expected that PCPs in the home-care hospice group would provide more hours of care to the dying patient than those in the hospital-based hospice group. This difference did prove to be significant (see chapter 7). One might then expect that the PCPs of HC patients would also feel the most burdened by the care they were providing during the period prior to the patient's death. This hypothesis was partially substantiated.

A seven-point feelings-of-burden scale was constructed to explore the extent to which the PCP was limited in other activities as a function of the amount of time spent in caring for the patient. This scale is based upon PCP self-reported responses given as part of the second interview (three or four weeks after study intake). The domains included are reduced social and leisure activities, strapped financial resources, and hindered ability to respond to other important needs. The score distributions on the feelings-of-burden scale are presented in table 9.9.

The hypothesis that felt burden would parallel actual expenditure of time and effort was supported in one instance (fig. 9.5). The PCPs of home-care hospice patients did express significantly higher feelings of burden than did the PCPs of hospital-based hospice patients. This finding is not at all surprising. What is interesting, however, is that the PCPs of home-care hospice patients do not score significantly higher than the PCPs of conventional-care patients. This indicates a positioning of the three samples with conventional care in the middle and implies that home-based hospices are particularly effective in reducing the feelings of burden that must to some extent accompany the strenuous efforts made by their PCPs.

The sense of burden appears to measure a vital component of the PCP's total life experience. Although felt burden does seem related to actual expenditure of caregiving effort, the situation is probably a good deal more complex. Why, for example, was the sense of burden not lower among PCPs associated with conventional-care programs? The differential effort required of the PCPs in CC and HC settings would appear to be rather great (as verified by reported hours of care given), yet the felt burden for the two groups is comparable.

Table 9.9   Percentage Distribution of Scores by Sample
for Feelings of Burden (by PCP) at PCP Follow-up Interview
Based on Three Questions

		CC	HB	HC
Most Burden	6	6.4	5.5	13.9
	5	11.0	9.1	14.3
	4	18.5	19.8	21.4
	3	16.8	17.0	20.1
	2	20.8	22.8	13.3
	1	12.0	15.2	8.7
Least Burden	0	14.5	10.6	8.3

Sample	Mean	Median	N
	2.71	2.66	173
	2.69	2.58	329
	3.36	3.48	482

Note: Scale developed by HRCA from Rand Corporation and HRCA items.

PCP responded at PCP follow-up interview to how much helping or caring for the patient:

Reduced social and leisure activities?
Strapped financial resources?
Hindered ability to respond to other important needs?

Extent of Bereavement Counseling

Does receiving bereavement counseling constitute a positive or negative outcome? It may be that the provision of appropriate supports to the PCP during the patient's terminal phase of life would eliminate the need for subsequent counseling services and also reduce the probability of a variety of other negative outcomes. On the other hand, bereavement counseling might be taken at face value as an index of stress and coping difficulties. The extent-of-bereavement-counseling measure used here includes assistance with financial matters and help in arranging for services as well as discussion of feelings. Not all the counseling interventions were directly related to anxiety, depression, and other responses to stress. A variety of life problems arose for PCPs during the three-month period from death to bereavement interview. Assistance with funeral arrangements, for example, seemed to be a frequent occasion for counseling in the broad sense of the term, and does not necessarily imply that the PCP was in emotional turmoil.

Approximately half of the PCPs across all three samples had either one concern that led to counseling or no such concerns (table 9.10). Relatively few PCPs sought counseling help in all five possible areas of concern (ranging across samples from 1.7 percent to 4.7 percent). Only about 9 percent of the PCPs (6 percent each in CC and HB, 12 percent in HC) received both interpersonal and legal/financing counseling. The adjusted impact findings presented

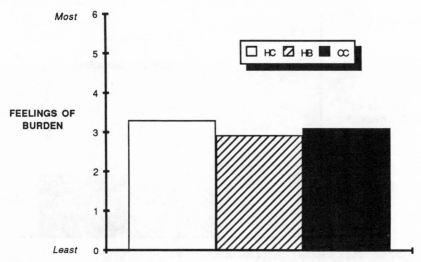

Figure 9.5   Mean Score on Feelings of Burden for PCP of "Average" Hospice Patient at Follow-up Interview

Table 9.10   Percentage Distribution of Scores by Sample for Extent of Bereavement Counseling (by PCP) since Pt's Death

		CC	HB	HC
Most Help	5	2.1	1.7	4.7
	4	2.9	4.4	8.1
	3	14.2	12.7	14.0
	2	22.1	23.6	24.9
	1	17.5	19.8	19.1
Least Help	0	41.3	37.8	29.3
Sample		Mean	Median	N
		1.26	1.00	240
		1.31	1.12	479
		1.67	1.57	680

Sum of positive responses to questions asked of PCP as to whether he or she had spoken with nonfamily members or friends about feelings, interpersonal problems, financial or legal assistance, or help securing services.

in figure 9.6 show that PCPs in the home-care hospice sample did receive significantly more counseling than either of the other two groups. It is possible that the home-based hospice's emphasis on bereavement counseling led to a more energetic reach-out program that contributed to the differential, but no data are available on this point.

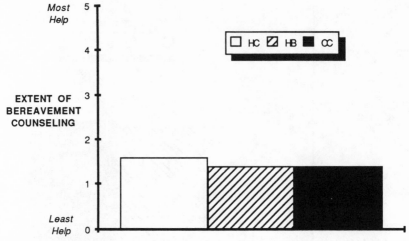

Figure 9.6   Mean Score on Extent of Bereavement Counseling for PCP of "Average" Hospice
Patient at Bereavement

PCP Dissatisfaction with Bereavement Counseling

The hospice emphasis suggested that PCPs of conventional-care patients would
be more dissatisfied with bereavement counseling (or its lack) than would PCPs
of hospice patients. Dissatisfaction with bereavement counseling (table 9.11)
was indicated if PCPs reported that they (1) did not have someone to turn to if
they had a question about how they were responding to the death, (2) were not
satisfied with the counseling and support they had received, or (3) wished that
they had made use of counseling services.

This hypothesis was not confirmed. Figure 9.7 shows that the adjusted
means for the PCPs are almost identical across the three care settings, with no
significant differences emerging. The PCPs of conventional-care patients did
not express more dissatisfaction with bereavement counseling or lack of bereavement counseling than did PCPs in the two types of hospice programs. It is
possible that those associated with conventional-care programs were in the

Table 9.11   Percentage Distribution of Scores by Sample for Dissatisfaction
with Bereavement Counseling (by PCP) at Bereavement Interview

	Score	CC	HB	HC
Dissatisfied	2	10.8	4.3	5.9
Not Dissatisfied	1	89.2	95.7	94.1
	Sample	Mean	Median	N
		1.11	1.06	259
		1.04	1.02	491
		1.06	1.03	714

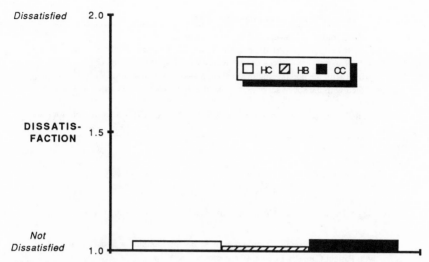

Figure 9.7   Mean Score on Dissatisfaction with Bereavement Counseling for PCP of "Average" Hospice Patient at Bereavement

position of people who are not likely to miss something they did not know even existed. Hospital care generally focuses upon the patient, and the obligation to offer bereavement counseling was placed upon participating hospice programs but not the participating hospitals. PCPs in conventional-care programs, then, may not have expected counseling and therefore did not miss what they did not receive.

Perhaps the most striking result is the almost universal lack of dissatisfaction with whatever bereavement counseling was received—a finding that does not explain anything but rather asks for further study.

Satisfaction with Patient Care

There was an expectation that PCPs of hospice patients would be more satisfied than PCPs of conventional-care patients with the health and supportive services provided to the patient in the last days of life. Furthermore, it was thought that PCPs of hospital-based hospice patients would be more satisfied than those of home-care hospice patients because pain control appeared to be the most effective in this type of program (chapter 7). These two outcomes were expected both when assessed during the terminal phase of illness and when reflected upon by the PCP during the bereavement interview. As will be seen below, these hypotheses were only partially supported by the data.

Satisfaction with patient care is based on PCP responses to questions relating to his or her overall satisfaction with both nursing/medical care and counseling services. It includes also the PCP's perception of the communication between

Table 9.12   Scoring of Satisfaction with Patient Care

PCP responded at initial, follow-up, and bereavement interview to:

The DOCTOR told ——— (Pt) all he or she WANTED to know about his or her illness.

The DOCTOR gave ——— (Pt) a chance to say what was really on his or her mind.

I was satisfied with the nursing and medical care ——— (Pt) received.

I was satisfied with the social services, counseling, and other support care ——— (Pt) received.

I was satisfied with the extent to which the DOCTORS and NURSES let me care for ——— (Pt).

Coding Options
Scale Recode
    0 = Disagree or Ambivalent
    0–2 = 2
    1 = Agree

Note: Scale developed by HRCA from Wolf, Rand Corporation, and HRCA items.

Table 9.13   Percentage Distribution of Scores by Sample for Satisfaction with Patient Care (by PCP) at Bereavement Interview

		CC	HB	HC
Most Satisfied	5	55.3	70.0	60.6
	4	25.1	17.5	20.5
	3	9.8	8.2	11.4
Least Satisfied	2	9.8	4.3	7.5
	Sample	Mean	Median	N
		4.26	4.60	235
		4.53	4.79	440
		4.34	4.67	664

Note: Scale developed by HRCA from Wolf, Rand Corporation, and HRCA items.

patient and physician and the PCP's satisfaction with his or her own opportunity to be involved in the care. (Scoring and frequency distributions are presented for all samples in tables 9.12 and 9.13.)

The findings indicate a rather high level of satisfaction with patient care for all three types of care programs. More than half of the PCPs in each sample score in the most-satisfied category. As figure 9.8 illustrates, the only significant difference in the adjusted mean satisfaction scores of PCPs across the three settings was in the comparison of the two hospice modalities. As hypothesized, the PCPs of hospital-based hospice patients were more satisfied than those of the home-care hospice patients. This differential holds true when assessed during the patient's life and when reflected upon by the PCP about three months after death.

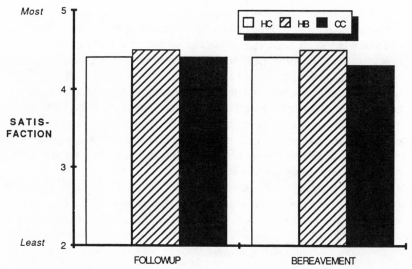

Figure 9.8   Mean Score on Satisfaction with Patient Care for PCP of "Average" Hospice Patient at Follow-up Interview and Bereavement

What Other Factors Are Related to Bereavement Outcome?

Up to this point the analysis of findings has focused on possible differences in bereavement outcome that could be attributed to the type of service provided (two hospice modalities and conventional care). This section now explores some of the other variables that might have been related to the primary care person's emotional, social, and physical status both during the terminal phase of the patient's life and in the first months of bereavement. The emphasis, then, is upon general relationships between the outcome variables and factors other than type of care provided. Of particular interest are three key bereavement outcomes: emotional stress, social reengagement, and number of physician visits.

Three questions were addressed by these exploratory analyses:

1. Can emotional stress, social reengagement, and physician visits be predicted by any of the information available at the time of study intake? In other words, can those at most risk for poor bereavement outcomes be identified early?

2. Do any of the preintervention variables correlate significantly with or predict all three key bereavement outcome measures across all three PCP samples?

3. To what extent are bereavement outcomes in different spheres of functioning correlated with each other across all three PCP samples?

The data utilized to explore the first two questions come from the zero-order correlational analyses derived in the course of creating the multivariate adjustments on relationship between study intake variables and the three key bereavement outcomes. Reported here are those preintervention variables that were found to be significantly related to poor outcomes in all three PCP samples. Additionally, differences within the PCP samples were examined for clues to the types of independent variables that might be predictive of high risk across all three PCP samples. This analysis involved statistical adjustments for differences among the three PCP samples at time of intake. The third question was examined through a zero-order correlation matrix of the larger set of outcome variables developed for each PCP sample.

A number of variables measured at the time of study intake did prove to have significant (.05 or lower) relationships with one or more of the bereavement outcome measures across all three samples. Variables showing significant relationships included sex, living arrangement, financial status, prior psychological and physical health status, and satisfaction with care. Specifically:

Sociodemographic Variables

Sex	Males are likely to have less social reengagement than are females during the first months of bereavement.
Living Arrangement	PCPs who live with the patient are likely to have more emotional stress and more doctor visits.
Financial Status	Income is inversely related to bereavement outcome: • PCPs with incomes under $5,000 are more likely to experience emotional stress during bereavement. • PCPs whose financial resources are reduced because of the care provided to the patient are more likely to experience emotional stress and have more doctor visits.
Education	PCPs with less education are likely to have more emotional stress during bereavement.
Marital Status	Emotional stress and doctor visits during bereavement were more likely if the PCP was married to the patient.
Child Status	PCPs who are children of the patient are less likely to have doctor visits during bereavement.
Age	Younger PCPs are less likely to have doctor visits during the bereavement period.

Social Supports

Family Tension	PCPs who are experiencing family tension at intake are likely to have more emotional stress at bereavement.

Psychological Characteristics at Study Intake

Mental Health — PCPs who were anxious or depressed were likely to have more emotional stress and more doctor visits at bereavement.

PCPs who had difficulty in sleeping were likely to have more emotional stress at bereavement.

PCPs who had headaches were likely to have more emotional stress at bereavement.

PCPs who required medication for "nerves" were likely to have more emotional stress and more doctor visits at bereavement.

PCPs who had experienced a change in weight were likely to have more emotional stress at bereavement.

PCPs who had cold sweats were likely to have more emotional stress at bereavement.

Coping Traits — PCPs who had feelings of burden were likely to have more emotional stress at bereavement.

PCPs who reduced their response to other needs because of caring for the patient were likely to have more emotional stress at bereavement.

Health Status at Study Intake

Wellness — PCPs who did not feel well most of the time were likely to have more emotional stress at bereavement.

PCPs who judged their health to be limited were likely to have more doctor visits at bereavement.

Energy — PCPs who reported not having plenty of energy at intake were more likely to experience emotional stress at bereavement.

Satisfaction with Care at Intake

Dissatisfied PCPs — PCPs who were dissatisfied with the care the patient was receiving at study intake were more likely than others to experience emotional stress at bereavement.

It can be seen that the same variables are not necessarily predictive of all three key bereavement outcomes (tables 9.14, 9.15, and 9.16). Poor physical and mental-health outcomes are more likely to be associated with emotional stress and doctor visits than with social reengagement.

Considered as a whole, two major propositions in the literature are clearly supported by the exploratory analyses: (1) spouses and persons in general who live with the patient are more likely to have poor physical and mental-health

Table 9.14 Correlations among Outcome Variables for PCP of CC Patients

	Emotional Stress at Bereavement	Number of Dr. Visits at Bereavement	Social Reengagement at Bereavement	Anxiety/ Depression at Follow-up	Feelings of Burden at Follow-up	Bereavement Counseling at Bereavement	Dissatisfactory Counseling at Bereavement	Satisfactory Pt Care at Bereavement
Emotional stress at bereavement								
Number of Dr. visits at bereavement	0.11 (220) $p = 0.083$							
Social reengagement at bereavement	0.07 (217) $p = 0.293$	.04 (257) $p = 0.473$						
Anxiety/depression at follow-up	0.38 (119) $p = <0.001$	0.00 (145) $p = 0.918$	0.22 (142) $p = 0.008$					
Feelings of burden at follow-up	0.27 (123) $p = 0.002$	0.05 (153) $p = 0.480$	0.09 (150) $p = 0.251$	0.38 (160) $p = <0.001$				
Bereavement counseling at bereavement	0.04 (219) $p = 0.504$	0.10 (240) $p = 0.094$	-0.01 (237) $p = 0.760$	0.08 (130) $p = 0.313$	0.17 (136) $p = 0.046$			
Dissatisfactory counseling at bereavement	0.35 (218) $p = <0.00$	-0.01 (258) $p = 0.869$	-0.03 (254) $p = 0.531$	0.18 (143) $p = 0.029$	0.14 (151) $p = 0.068$	-0.07 (239) $p = 0.231$		
Satisfactory Pt Care at bereavement	0.06 (200) $p = 0.364$	0.04 (232) $p = 0.485$	-0.07 (229) $p = 0.251$	-0.12 (129) $p = 0.154$	-0.00 (137) $p = 0.976$	0.07 (216) $p = 0.285$	-0.07 (230) $p = 0.265$	

Table 9.15 Correlations among Outcome Variables for PCP of HB Patients

	Emotional Stress at Bereavement	Number of Dr. Visits at Bereavement	Social Reengagement at Bereavement	Anxiety/ Depression at Follow-up	Feelings of Burden at Follow-up	Bereavement Counseling at Bereavement	Dissatisfactory Counseling at Bereavement	Satisfactory Pt Care at Bereavement
Emotional stress at bereavement								
Number of Dr. visits at bereavement	0.26 (425) $p = <0.001$							
Social reengagement at bereavement	0.02 (402) $p = 0.372$	-0.04 (472) $p = 0.203$						
Anxiety/depression at follow-up	0.44 (226) $p = <0.001$	0.20 (264) $p = 0.001$	0.107 (252) $p = 0.044$					
Feelings of burden at follow-up	0.23 (235) $p = <0.001$	0.11 (273) $p = 0.036$	0.04 (260) $p = 0.277$	0.46 (318) $p = <0.000$				
Bereavement counseling at bereavement	0.23 (423) $p = <0.001$	0.19 (479) $p = <0.001$	0.40 (458) $p = 0.014$	-0.08 (256) $p = 0.094$	-0.04 (265) $p = 0.253$			
Dissatisfactory counseling at bereavement	0.16 (420) $p = <0.001$	-0.01 (491) $p = 0.383$	-0.03 (486) $p = 0.267$	0.19 (262) $p = 0.001$	-0.14 (271) $p = 0.009$	-0.00 (473) $p = 0.488$		
Satisfactory Pt Care at bereavement	-0.08 (377) $p = 0.053$	0.02 (440) $p = 0.357$	0.06 (417) $p = 0.900$	-0.12 (239) $p = 0.029$	-0.11 (246) $p = 0.039$	0.01 (423) $p = 0.391$	-0.02 (437) $p = 0.358$	

Table 9.16 Correlations among Outcome Variables for PCP of HC Patients

	Emotional Stress at Bereavement	Number of Dr. Visits at Bereavement	Social Reengagement at Bereavement	Anxiety/ Depression at Follow-up	Feelings of Burden at Follow-up	Bereavement Counseling at Bereavement	Dissatisfactory Counseling at Bereavement	Satisfactory Pt Care at Bereavement
Emotional stress at bereavement								
Number of Dr. visits at bereavement	0.30 (620) $p = <0.001$							
Social reengagement at bereavement	−0.06 (603) $p = 0.482$	0.06 (731) $p = 0.058$						
Anxiety/depression at follow-up	0.46 (372) $p = <0.001$	0.15 (426) $p = 0.001$	0.11 (415) $p = 0.010$					
Feelings of burden at follow-up	0.19 (374) $p = <0.001$	0.10 (433) $p = 0.027$	0.10 (421)	0.36 (470) $p = <0.001$				
Bereavement counseling at bereavement	0.20 (616) $p = <0.001$	0.12 (680) $p = 0.001$	0.04 (660) $p = 0.179$	0.02 (405) $p = 0.347$	−0.05 (408) $p = 0.136$			
Dissatisfactory counseling at bereavement	0.19 (615) $p = <0.001$	0.08 (714) $p = 0.022$	−0.07 (692) $p = 0.029$	0.14 (421) $p = 0.002$	0.05 (426) $p = 0.162$	−0.05 (674) $p = 0.101$		
Satisfactory Pt Care at bereavement	−0.07 (576) $p = 0.053$	0.01 (664) $p = 0.476$	−0.00 (698) $p = 0.484$	−0.11 (398) $p = 0.015$	−0.14 (404) $p = 0.003$	−0.02 (624) $p = 0.325$	−0.14 (659) $p = <0.001$	

182

outcomes; and (2) poor mental and physical health on the part of the PCP while the patient is still living is predictive of poor mental health (as measured by emotional stress) during the early months of bereavement. The mental-health indices seem to be especially powerful predictors, although it should be noted that some of these items include somatic manifestations such as headaches and cold sweats.

These characteristics that exist at intake, however, do not predict the extent to which social reengagement will occur during the first months of bereavement. The degree to which the PCP's social activities were curtailed during the terminal phase of the patient's life appears to be the most useful predictor. Social reengagement also seems to be a domain of functioning that is relatively independent of emotional stress, at least during the early period of bereavement studied here. It is possible that several different types of functional relationships may be operating. Some people may have a temporary but strong need for "time out" from interpersonal obligations. Family members have told us of the craving for "quiet time," and "getting back to myself and seeing where I am now." Other former PCPs may take advantage of the renewed opportunity for social involvement, but not necessarily to relieve emotional stress. Social activities can serve to fill time, provide outlets for energy, and restore the individual's sense of being part of a larger community. Still other individuals may seek social reengagement primarily as a way to reduce emotional distress and loneliness. Although social reengagement is an important component of the individual's total life situation, it does not seem to have a simple relationship with emotional stress.

Conclusion

The first months of bereavement will be difficult for most people. The analyses reported in this chapter attempted to determine whether or not variations in type of service (two hospice modalities and conventional care) had an influence on the level and pattern of difficulty experienced by those who had served as principal care persons for a loved one. We also tried to identify some characteristics of the PCP and the situation that might provide early warning signs for those at greatest risk to experience especially poor bereavement outcomes.

The impact analysis can perhaps be summarized best through a combined hypothesis that formulates the major advantages attributed to the hospice approach: *Differences in bereavement outcomes will be observed as a function of the generic program (hospital-based hospice, home-care hospice, or conventional care) to which the patient and PCP are exposed, with the most beneficial outcomes generally expected for PCPs served by hospital-based and home care–based hospice programs.*

As it turned out, National Hospice Study findings only partially support this overall hypothesis. The only significant difference between conventional care and the hospice modalities was in the area of bereavement counseling. Furthermore, this finding lends itself to alternative explanations—the more frequent use of counseling (in the broad sense of the term) by PCPs in the home-care hospice setting could represent either a response to heightened feelings of burden and emotional distress or the result of more extensive reach-out efforts by the home-care agencies. An advantage for the PCPs of home-care patients seems to exist in their higher levels of reported social reengagement. This shift, however, might simply represent a return to prior social activities after a period of intensive activities centering around the terminally ill family member.

The PCPs of hospital-based hospice patients fared significantly better than those of home-based hospice patients with respect to emotional stress, feelings of burden, and satisfaction with patient care both before and after the death of the patient. On these key variables the three samples are positioned with hospital-based hospice care at the top or "best" position and home-care hospice care jockeying with conventional care or more often in the "low" position with respect to specific variables. This pattern of findings is consistent with the quality-of-life data (chapter 7), in which patients in hospital-based hospice programs had significantly lower levels of pain and other symptoms. To the extent that impact differences can be demonstrated, then, the hospital-based hospice program emerges in the most positive light.

Several points should be kept in mind, however, before drawing firm conclusions: (1) The hospice movement is still relatively new and continues to learn from its experiences; (2) Conventional-care programs have not been impervious to the innovations introduced by the hospice movement; and (3) Some of the most important determinants of bereavement outcome are related to characteristics of the patient, the PCP, and the total family situation, rather than to the particular type of care program provided. All three types of programs might be able to reduce negative bereavement outcomes even more successfully if those at particular risk were identified at intake. Some of the information provided by the exploratory analyses reported in this chapter could prove valuable in this endeavor—for example, the relatively greater risk for PCPs who are married to the terminally ill patient and for PCPs who have a number of psychosomatic problems of their own. Although HB, HC, and CC programs might take somewhat different courses of action, all could find ways to provide additional support and stress-reduction measures to those at greatest risk for poor bereavement outcomes.

Furthermore, expectations regarding bereavement outcome deserve careful review. How realistic is it to expect any terminal-care program to have a strong and consistent impact on bereavement outcome? Despite important differences among the three approaches studied here, it is likely that all have much in common. Physicians and nurses, for example, may be just as competent across all three settings. Increased sensitivity to the social and emotional needs of terminally ill people may have affected the performance of staff in conventional care as well as in hospice programs. It is also likely that grief in response to bereavement is only one of the processes that have a major effect on subsequent mood and coping ability. Fatigue, "burnout," financial problems, and other factors associated with an arduous period of providing care should not be neglected and do, in fact, show up in the NHS findings. Another significant characteristic shared by PCPs in all three groups was knowledge of the patient's limited life expectancy. If anticipatory grief is as important as many researchers and clinicians believe, then this process probably was active among PCPs in all three samples, thereby perhaps exercising more influence than some of the variables associated with differential care programs.

Three alternative general hypotheses were offered earlier in this chapter. Examined now in light of the findings, one can see that the hospice approach does place a heavier burden on the primary care person, especially when much of the care is provided in the home setting. This does not necessarily mean, however, that this form of care should be discouraged. It simply reminds us that all forms of caring exact a price. We would not grieve if we did not love. The NHS focus on the first months of bereavement may have captured feelings of stress and burden at or near their peak. At a later period the same former PCPs may have recuperated their energies and retained the long-term sense of satisfaction in having given so much of themselves to a loved one. The second hypothesis proposed that bereavement outcomes should be less negative for those enrolled in hospice programs because the relationship between PCP and patient would receive the most support and the least disruption. The fact that patients enrolled in home-care hospice programs did in fact spend more time at home provides objective support for one component of the hypothesis. The impact findings, however, do not demonstrate an overall superiority in alleviating the PCPs' distress during the early months of bereavement. The most satisfactory way to determine why this part of the hypothesis was not supported would be to conduct new studies designed more specifically to analyze *process* as well as outcome. Provisionally, we might consider the possibilities, such as (1) some PCPs *prefer* that the medical establishment take the leading role in provision of care, and (2) protection of the PCP/patient relationship may be important but not as differentially important in affecting bereavement outcomes as other factors involved in the situation (e.g., energy outlay required of the PCP). The third hypothesis suggested that most people adjust to whatever situations exist, therefore this adaptive capacity on the part of the PCPs will take precedence over the particularities of each program type. This hypothesis draws indirect support from the fact that most PCPs in all three settings expressed a high degree of satisfaction with patient care. More direct and extensive examination of this hypothesis might prove fruitful in the future and possibly provide a corrective for the tendency to assume that program variations necessarily make a difference.

Although the NHS analysis of bereavement outcomes was intended primarily as a comparative evaluation of three program types, perhaps the data can be utilized most productively in helping all those involved in terminal care in the continuing challenge to improve their services. There is nothing in the NHS data that points clearly to the abandonment of either hospice modality or conventional care. That all three programs exist is a definite advantage for those patients, family members, and health-care professionals who wish to exercise their options and make knowledgeable choices.

10

The Hospice Volunteer

LINDA LALIBERTE
AND VINCENT MOR

Volunteers have played a major role in both the emergence and the development of individual hospices. This involvement provided the momentum for the movement to recognize, accept, and incorporate the hospice philosophy into the existing health-care system. The individual and joint efforts of these volunteers have contributed to the transformation of hospice care from a little-known and unreimbursed service to a widely recognized alternative form of treatment for terminally ill patients and their families. It is largely because of their commitment that the hospice movement was able to gain this recognition.

This chapter examines a number of issues related to the use of volunteers in hospices during a period of organizational evolvement and, in some cases, growth. Following a brief discussion of the role of volunteerism in the development of the hospice movement and individual hospices, we describe the volunteers and their activities, the relationship of third-party reimbursement and hospice organizational structure to the level of volunteer activities, and, finally, what may lie ahead for the hospice volunteer as a result of the introduction of reimbursement.

NHS data are used to compare the demographic composition of volunteers in the three major hospice organizational types—hospital-affiliated (HAF), freestanding (FRE), and home health agency–based (HHA). We examine the attitudes of paid staff toward volunteers and the factors that motivate the volunteers to work in the hospice. The types of activities performed by volunteers are compared across the three organizational types. In particular, we examine the proportion of time spent in patient-care activities compared to administrative activities. One might expect that hospices that are not affiliated with an institution would utilize volunteers for administrative support to a greater degree than the hospital- or home health agency–affiliated organizations. One might also expect that with the introduction of third-party reimbursement, the use of volunteers to provide care to patients will diminish and that volunteers will ultimately be replaced by paid staff. These and other questions are explored in this chapter.

Background

Many of the earliest hospices began entirely as volunteer efforts. The inhumane treatment of the terminally ill was identified as a health-care problem. Through the initiative of dedicated individuals, an attempt was made to develop a solution that would meet the needs of the patients. In the case of Hospice, Inc. of New Haven, Connecticut, the process began with the formation of committees, research teams, and task forces. Like-minded professionals and community leaders met in these forums to develop a model for the care of the dying, a model based upon St. Christopher's Hospice in London (Stoddard 1978). Through the efforts of these volunteers, funding was obtained, the community relations were defined, and the hospice concept was established with local health and human service providers. In 1973, Hospice, Inc. became the first American hospice.

Volunteerism in the pioneer hospices was manifested in two main areas: (1) a voluntary board of directors, composed usually of health professionals with community linkages; and (2) a voluntary labor force to provide services to patients and their families. The use of a community board of directors capitalized not only on professional expertise, but also provided a network with the capability of raising funds, recruiting additional volunteers, and assisting and promoting the hospice's development. This model affirmed the hospice's legitimacy in the community, served as an efficient public relations resource, and created an image of community partnership (Paradis 1983). A voluntary labor force was essential in many of the early hospices, since the services were not covered by third parties. Hospices had to keep their labor costs low in order to survive. In many instances, the community board and the voluntary labor force consisted of the same core of dedicated individuals.

While these volunteer origins are common to the three main hospice organizational types, there are differences inherent to these organizations that may affect the integration of the volunteer and the substance of his or her responsibility. Since FRE hospices lack institutional affiliation and support, they presumably rely upon volunteers to fill diverse roles to a greater degree than HAF or HHA hospices. Staff in HAF hospices are accustomed to the use of volunteers to augment the care they provide and to fill a variety of nonpatient care roles (e.g., gift shop, reception desk). While hospice volunteers assume greater "hands-on" responsibility for patient care, HAF hospice staff may find the transition to volunteer-provider easier than HHA hospices, which have not traditionally used volunteers in any capacity. NHS data are used to compare the hospice volunteer across these three organizational types to gain some insight into the incorporation and use of this growing labor force into both established and developing organizations.

The NHS was undertaken to evaluate the quality and cost of hospice care and to examine organizational characteristics related to the rapid growth experienced by hospices following the introduction of Medicare reimbursement under the HCFA demonstration. With regard to the volunteer component of hospice organizations, we hypothesized a priori that the use of volunteers to deliver direct patient services would decrease with the availability of reimbursement (Greer et al. 1983). Our rationale was that paid professional staff would be substituted for volunteer staff to provide those services that were reimbursable and that volunteers would be assigned new roles within the organization. As will be seen in this chapter, the data did not support this hypothesis.

Who Is the Hospice Volunteer?

Historically, volunteers have most often contributed their time to health and human service agencies. The hospice volunteer differs in significant respects from most earlier models of the volunteer. Although still most often a female, the hospice volunteer is not to be confused with either the "Lady Bountifuls" or the "candy stripers" whose activities created the stereotype of the volunteer. The middle-aged woman from an affluent background and the teenage girl provided services of a peripheral and supplemental nature. Welcome as these services might have been, they were not considered part of the basic therapeutic plan. There was a sharp distinction between professional and volunteer, with the latter entrusted only with services eschewed by the former.

Another type of previous model was that of the community business leader who served on the board of a voluntary agency. This community link provided valuable public relations and support, but rarely were the dual functions of direct service and public relations provided by the same individual.

By contrast, many key figures in the hospice movement integrated both the therapeutic and administrative functions. Furthermore, unlike the candy striper or Lady Bountiful, those helping to establish hospice systems often had professional qualifications in health-related fields. Those contributing their services on a volunteer basis to hospices, then, are part of a newer tradition, one in which substantial clinical and/or operational responsibilities are entrusted. This, in turn, may be seen as part of a larger break from the previous tradition that also includes trained volunteers serving in suicide prevention centers and a variety of other counseling situations.

Survey Results

As part of the routine NHS data collection, an anonymous staff questionnaire was administered to all paid and volunteer staff at each of the participating hospices. There were no significant differences in the demographic composition of volunteers across the three organizational types. As can be seen in table 10.1, most volunteers were female, white, middle-aged, and educated beyond the high school level. This makeup is consistent with the typical picture of Lady Bountifuls in community services, and, with the exception of the candy striper model, is consistent with hospital volunteers as well. The modal family income for volunteers surveyed was over $30,000 across all three hospice types, considerably higher than that of the generally elderly patient population served.

There is significant anecdotal and other evidence to suggest that many hospice volunteers are health-care professionals. We were told of many instances in which nurses would complete their regular shifts and then visit

Table 10.1   Demographics of Hospice Volunteers by Type of Hospice

| | Percentage | | | |
Demographics	Home Health Agency (N = 65)	Freestanding (N = 156)	Hospital-Affiliated (N = 112)	Total (N = 333)
Sex				
Male	12.3	13.5	12.5	12.9
Female	75.4	78.2	75.0	76.6
Missing	12.3	8.3	12.5	10.5
Race/Ethnicity				
White	84.6	91.0	87.5	88.6
Nonwhite	3.1	0.6	0.0	0.9
Hispanic	3.1	1.9	0.9	1.8
Non-Hispanic	84.6	90.4	85.7	87.7
Missing	12.3	8.3	12.5	10.5
Education				
< High School	13.8	18.6	20.5	18.3
High School +	76.9	72.4	64.3	70.6
Missing	9.2	9.0	15.2	11.1
Family Income				
<$10,000	3.1	9.6	14.3	9.9
$10,000–$20,000	12.3	26.9	21.4	22.2
$20,001–$30,000	15.4	19.9	16.1	17.7
$30,000+	50.8	30.1	29.5	33.9
Missing	18.5	13.5	18.8	16.2
Age				
18–40	32.3	32.1	35.7	33.3
41–64	49.2	44.2	36.6	42.6
65+	6.2	12.2	13.4	11.4
Missing	12.3	11.5	14.3	12.6

hospice patients, and of "retired" social workers or nurses who conducted volunteer training sessions in addition to carrying their patient caseload. Given the active role of volunteers in the development of hospices, this information was not surprising, and it certainly affirmed that hospice volunteers were different from their Lady Bountiful and candy striper counterparts. As will be seen below, this difference is apparent in the activities of the hospice volunteer.

What motivates these individuals to become hospice volunteers? Our survey indicated that over 87 percent were motivated by interest in the hospice movement, but nearly 84 percent of volunteers were motivated by the opportunity for career advancement. When viewed with the demographic characteristics of hospice volunteers, this finding suggests that the hospice may be serving a function for women who have decided to join or reenter the work force after raising their families, for health-care providers interested in changing careers, and for individuals seeking self-fulfillment. It is a stepping stone in the sense that it provides training and development of skills that may be marketable to other areas of the same hospice organization, to other developing hospices, or to the human service system in general. There is anecdotal evidence suggesting the key position of hospice volunteer director or coordinator is increasingly becoming a paid position, and it is frequently offered to a hospice volunteer.

A recent study of volunteers at Mercy Hospice Care Program, Urbana, Illinois, provides a useful comparison with the NHS survey. Patchner and Finn (1987–88) also found that most of the volunteers (93 percent) were female, white (84 percent), and married (63 percent). Also similar to volunteers surveyed by NHS, those in Urbana tended to be educated beyond the high school level (65 percent with college backgrounds). Almost all the Urbana volunteers (95 percent) considered themselves to be in good or excellent health, and many (57 percent) were active in other volunteer activities as well, often centering around their churches. Almost one of five (19 percent) were employed in a health-service field, and another 21 percent in education. The most frequently expressed motivation for becoming a hospice volunteer (44 percent) was simply to "be of service to others," while another 18 percent felt that hospice care was an especially needed program. Other expressed motives were divided among many categories, with only 9 percent citing career-related reasons.

Using a modified version of the Maslach burnout inventory (Maslach 1976), we compared the attitudes of hospice volunteers and paid staff. They were asked to apply ratings (never, rarely, sometimes, often, always) to a series of statements. Factor analysis of their responses yielded three reliable subscales: emotional exhaustion, personal accomplishment, and depersonalization.

When the relationship between these three scales and the variable volunteer status was examined, volunteers scored significantly lower on the emotional exhaustion and depersonalization scales than paid staff, but they did not differ from paid staff members with respect to feelings of personal accomplishment (Mor and Laliberte 1984). This finding may reflect the more time-limited in-

Table 10.2   Staff Attitudes toward Volunteers by Type of Hospice

	Percentage				
	Home Health Agency (N = 229)	Freestanding (N = 197)	Hospital-Affiliated (N = 269)	Total (N = 695)	Degree of Significance
Helpful in Providing Moral Support to Patients					
Yes	87.2	85.9	94.1	89.5	.01
No	12.8	14.1	5.9	10.5	
Helpful in Providing Direct Patient Care					
Yes	48.5	58.4	56.1	54.2	.1
No	51.5	41.6	43.9	45.8	
Helpful in Performing Administrative Tasks					
Yes	23.6	64.2	37.9	62.1	<.001
No	76.4	35.8	62.1	40.8	
Helpful in Saving Staff Time					
Yes	51.5	74.8	71.3	65.9	<.001
No	48.5	25.2	28.7	34.1	
Helpful Often					
Yes	88.1	95.0	92.9	91.6	.05
No	11.9	5.0	7.1	8.1	

volvement of volunteers, which may reduce the sense of anxiety and pressure felt by paid staff who are responsible for carrying out the program.

In many cases, hospice volunteers deliver patient services that are not substantially different from the services delivered by paid staff. This pattern was also found by Patchner and Finn (1987–88). In order to gain insight into the integration of this additional class of providers into the organization, we examined staff perceptions of volunteer roles. In the NHS questionnaire, paid staff answered several items regarding volunteers' helpfulness. Contrary to reports of resistance of paid professional staff toward volunteers in human service programs (Haeuser and Schwartz 1980), the response of paid hospice staff was overwhelmingly positive. These data are presented in table 10.2. Staff in HHA hospices were less positive in their assessment of volunteers' helpfulness. This is most marked in the response to "helpful in saving staff time," suggesting that volunteers as a new phenomenon in an HHA are not as integrated into the organization's structure. Rather, their introduction constituted an entirely new development for HHAs. As was seen in chapter 2, there are fewer volunteers in HHA hospices. These numbers alone could suggest less visibility to paid staff and a less marked perception of helpfulness among paid staff. On the other hand, HAF staff were more likely to view volunteers as "helpful in providing moral support to patients." This is consistent with the traditional view of the volunteer role in a hospital setting. Finally, FRE staff viewed volunteers not only as extensions in providing patient care, but they also valued volunteers for their administrative contribution in FRE hospices. We shall see below that this attitudinal difference is reflected in the roles volunteers actually fill across these three hospice types.

The Activities of the Hospice Volunteer

Although the demographic composition of volunteers did not vary according to the hospice organizational structure, HAF, HHA, and FRE hospices might be expected to utilize volunteer labor differently. Volunteer activities are described in this section and compared across the three organizational types.

Throughout the study, monthly summaries reporting the number of hours spent by volunteers in hospice activities were routinely gathered. We classified volunteer activity as "direct patient care," which includes time spent with patients in an inpatient setting or during a home visit, and "administrative," which is other time not spent with patients. For a twelve-month period, we compared the proportion of time volunteers spent in direct patient care and administrative activities as a function of the availability of Medicare reimbursement for hospice services and a function of the hospice's organizational structure.

While the overall level of volunteer involvement was nearly the same in demonstration and nondemonstration hospices, we found substantial differences in the proportion of time spent in patient care and administrative activities as a function of the availability of reimbursement. Volunteers in nondemonstration hospices spent 70 percent of their time in patient-care activities as compared to only 43.2 percent in demonstration hospices. We confirmed the probability that these findings were indicative of a true difference by subjecting them to statistical analysis. Using a two-way analysis of variance on the weighted average of the proportion of patient-care time spent by volunteers, we found that the degree of patient-care activity was significantly related to the hospice's demonstration status. It should be pointed out that the unit of analysis here is the hospice. With only thirty-nine cases under investigation, any difference associated with demonstration status or organizational type would have to be very large before statistical significance could be observed. Consequently, a probability value of 0.10 was accepted as significant for facility-level analyses. Contrary to our findings with regard to patient-care activities, the proportion of volunteer time spent in administrative activities was not related to demonstration status. Possibly these findings are associated with a low volunteer rate among professional administrators.

The proportion of time volunteers spent in patient-care activities also differed by hospice organizational structure. We found that HAF hospices used over 70 percent of their volunteer time for patient-care activities. (Two-thirds of this time was spent in an inpatient setting.) HHA and FRE hospice volunteers spent about 50 percent and 41 percent, respectively, of their time in patient-care activities. Freestanding hospices, which began as volunteer-dominated organizations, used three to four times as many volunteer hours as either HAF or HHA hospices. The proportion of time spent in administrative activities at these FRE sites was higher than HHA or HAF hospices, indicating that FRE sites that have no institutional affiliation relied more heavily on their volunteers to assist with administrative activities, while HAF and HHA hospices may have utilized their affiliate's existing administrative resources such as personnel, purchasing, and billing. Results of a two-way analysis of variance confirm that there was a significant difference in the proportion of time spent by volunteers in both patient care ($p = .001$) and administrative activities ($p = 0.066$) as a function of organizational structure. As with many measures of hospice behavior presented in this chapter, the averages belie considerable heterogeneity among participating hospices. Tables 10.3 and 10.4 present site-specific averages concerning the total number of volunteer hours and the number of direct-care volunteer hours per month available to each site. These site-specific data indicate that FRE hospices are the more volunteer-oriented organizations.

Bereavement follow-up services have been an important facet of hospice care from the beginning. This service generally has been provided by volunteers. Although systematic evaluation of bereavement care is lacking, hospice experts believe that volunteers often provide sensitive and effective services in this area. Zimmerman (1981), for example, observes that volunteers are often

Table 10.3 A Comparison of Services Performed by Volunteers in Hospital-affiliated, Freestanding, and Home Health Agency Hospices (average total volunteer hours)

Service	HAF	FRE	HHA	Total	
				n	%
Art, Music Therapy	3.3	5.1	6.8	37	5.0
Bereavement Services	6.5	9.3	4.2	53	7.1
Continuous Home Care	0.8	2.6	2.6	15	2.0
Continuous Nursing	1.2	0.0	0.5	4	0.5
Day Care	6.9	0.6	0.0	19	2.5
Home Health Services	1.6	4.5	5.3	28	3.7
Homemaking Services	1.6	0.3	8.9	22	2.9
Nutritional, Occupational, or Physical Therapy	0.4	0.9	0.0	4	0.5
Recreation Therapy	0.8	0.3	0.5	4	0.5
Respite Care	0.4	8.3	10.5	47	6.3
Skilled Nursing	6.9	9.9	12.1	71	9.5
Social Services	2.9	9.0	6.3	47	6.3
Transportation	4.1	7.4	4.2	41	5.5
Other	62.4	41.7	37.9	354	47.5

Table 10.4   Distribution of Volunteer Activities
Reported during Patient Visits

Activity	Percentage
Companionship	38.2
Emotional Counseling	21.1
Assessment/Evaluation	7.7
Patient Care	6.3
Personal Care	6.2
Housekeeping	5.2
Patient/Family Education	4.9
Symptom Control	4.0
Pain Control	2.4
Financial/Legal Counseling	1.2
Referral	1.1
Supervision	1.1
Attendance at Death	0.6
TOTAL	100.0

in a better position to provide direct services than are other members of the hospice-care team. The volunteer is "often seen by the patient and his family as someone outside the normal health-care-delivery system and they are thus sometimes willing to share thoughts and feelings which they do not wish to express to other members of the team" (Zimmerman 1981, 110). For bereavement counseling, volunteers are considered to be especially valuable, representing the continued interest and support of the community and often drawing upon their own experiences with the loss of a loved one. Volunteers largely created the role of bereavement counseling; therefore, the fact that this service is generally still nonreimbursable may not represent a significant problem, as volunteers seem to remain the provider of choice for this service in most instances.

The HCFA demonstration did provide reimbursement for up to three bereavement visits. Volunteers reported spending approximately 20 hours per month in the provision of bereavement services. This figure represented 6.2 percent of their patient-care time in demonstration sites and 10.7 percent in nondemonstration hospices, suggesting that the availability of reimbursement was not a critical factor. This finding may indicate that bereavement programs will continue to remain the province of volunteers.

Volunteers clearly spend a great deal of time with hospice patients, but what happens during this time? On a series of random days throughout the study, we asked paid and volunteer staff to complete a log documenting their activities. Approximately 750 volunteer visits were analyzed to determine the kinds of activities that took place. Volunteers were asked first to classify the purpose of the visit. As can be seen in table 10.3, most visits fall into the "other" category, indicating that volunteers may be augmenting patient and family care, that is, meeting those needs that are not addressed by health-care providers. Skilled-nursing visits did account for 9.5 percent of the volunteer visits in the sample. This service was provided less frequently by HAF volunteers than by volunteers in the other two hospice types. The opposite was observed for day-care services, which were provided almost exclusively by HAF volunteers. These findings may reflect the differences in treatment setting across the three hospice types. Since HAF hospices use more inpatient care, there may be less need for skilled-nursing visits and more need for day care. Across all three hospices, over 30 percent of reported visits, volunteers provided art/music therapy, bereavement services, social services, respite care, or transportation.

Volunteers were next asked to identify which activities were performed during the visit. They were asked to record up to three activities that characterized the nature of the visit. As can be seen in table 10.4, companionship and emotional counseling were most often provided to hospice patients and their families. However, there were frequently multiple activities taking place during single visits. For the approximately 750 visits in our sample, volunteers reported being engaged in 1,395 activities. The range of patient-care activities performed by the hospice volunteer suggests that she or he may be in the best position to serve the varied and complex needs of patients and families experiencing terminal illness.

Although the majority of volunteer time was devoted to patients, a considerable amount of time was dedicated to administrative activities. We did not collect specific data on the types of administrative activities performed, but anecdotal evidence indicates that volunteers served in many capacities, from clerk/receptionist to fund-raiser. Volunteers assisted in the recruitment, selection, and training of new volunteers. They advocated for patients, and they promoted hospice care in many forums; they met with community groups, politicians, and members of the health-care professions.

The "administrative" activities described here go beyond the tasks performed by hospice volunteers during their weekly ten-hour commitment. In addition to providing patient care and serving in an administrative capacity, volunteers have an important role as private citizens, advocating for the delivery of humane services to those in need and sharing their enthusiasm for this innovative service with the community. This continued grass-roots involvement in the hospice movement has helped to assure that it remain true to its philosophy. The presence of a corps of volunteers has helped reduce the risk of over-bureaucratization and alienation that sometimes accompanies the formalization of a new health service. These volunteers may also be viewed as the conscience of the movement. With no vested interest in reimbursement or continued employment, they may be in the best position to keep the hospice true to its goals.

Changes in the Magnitude of Volunteer Involvement

We examined the level of volunteer involvement over a twelve-month period to determine whether any shifts occurred and whether these shifts were related to the availability of reimbursement or to the hospice organizational structure.

Number of Volunteer Hours

The number of hours spent by hospice volunteers was examined over twelve months to determine whether there was a relationship between the availability of reimbursement (demonstration status) and the level of volunteer involvement. The total number of volunteer hours per month was comparable for demonstration and nondemonstration sites, with nondemonstration hospices showing a slight decrease over time. The same data examined by organizational type showed that the level of volunteer activity in FRE hospices was four times greater than in either HHA or HAF hospices.

Analysis of variance on the number of volunteer hours per month averaged over the twelve months revealed no significant difference by demonstration status. A highly significant difference was found among the three organizational types on the twelve-month average. Across all sites an overall time effect ($p = 0.045$) was obtained, which appeared to be related to fluctuations and not reflective of a consistent trend. No differential change in the number of volunteer hours was observed over the twelve months as a function of demonstration status, organizational type, or an interaction of both. Thus, all hospices utilized a relatively constant level of volunteers throughout the course of the study. As will be seen in the next chapter, the relatively constant level of volunteer use is in contrast to substantial increases in the number of patients admitted and the number of new staff hired, particularly in FRE and HHA hospices.

The discrepancy between growth in hospice patient load and a steady level of volunteer use suggests that hospices may have had insufficient time to devote to the recruitment, training, and supervision of additional volunteers. Perhaps this is due in part to the administrative burden of study participation and rapid growth. However, it is more likely a function of each individual hospice's staffing plan. Following recruitment and screening, volunteers require training and supervision. Only a finite number of hospice staff hours may be available for these tasks—particularly supervision, which is an ongoing activity the inadequacy of which could have serious effects on patients, volunteers, and the hospices themselves. We may be observing the saturation point for the number of volunteer hours that may be effectively utilized and safely managed by hospice organizations. After assessing their staffing needs, hospices may devote only those resources necessary to maintain an appropriate level of volunteer activity. On the other hand, particularly among demonstration hospices, with the availability of funding, the hospices may have found it easier to hire new staff rather than invest in volunteers.

Volunteer Hours per Patient Day

Demonstration hospices served more patients than nondemonstration hospices, and the average number of admissions per quarter showed a marked increase during the study period. To examine shifts in volunteer use, it was necessary to adjust for differences in the size and differential rates of growth of hospices in the sample. This was accomplished by dividing the number of volunteer hours by the number of patients in the hospice on an average day for that period—a patient day.

There was a twofold difference in the number of volunteer hours per patient day by demonstration status. Demonstration hospice volunteers were available an average of 0.47 hours per patient day, compared to approximately 0.95 hours in nondemonstration sites. FRE volunteers devoted an average of 1.0 hours per patient day compared to approximately 0.50 hours and 0.27 hours in HAF and HHA hospices, respectively.

Further statistical analyses revealed a significant demonstration by organizational type interaction ($p = 0.094$). This suggests that organizational types are behaving differently depending on their demonstration status. A review of the data revealed that the average number of volunteer hours per patient day in FRE nondemonstration hospices was 2.0, compared to 0.65 in FRE demonstration sites. Clearly, much of the difference observed for organizational type appears to be attributable to the nondemonstration FRE hospices, suggesting that the availability of Medicare reimbursement may have allowed demonstration FRE hospices, all of which began as volunteer movements, to "replace" volunteers with paid staff. Indeed, the changes may have begun before the NHS; having been selected, these hospices hired additional staff and began to serve more patients.

The number of volunteer hours per patient day was examined across the twelve-month study period to determine whether any shifts were occurring over time in demonstration and nondemonstration hospices. Repeated measures analysis of variance revealed no overall time effect across all sites. A highly significant differential change was observed as a function of demonstration status ($p < 0.001$). Nondemonstration hospices, particularly FRE sites, experienced greater fluctuations and reductions in volunteer activity per patient day compared to the more stable levels of volunteer involvement evidenced in demonstration sites. This finding suggested that the level of volunteer involvement in nondemonstration sites may have been less responsive to shifts in patient census. Because of their small size, relatively small changes in census cause large shifts in volunteer hours per patient day. Statistical analyses reveal no significant differential change over time for the three organizational types.

The data do suggest that each organizational type may reach a different level of equilibrium, with HHA hospices providing fewer volunteer hours per patient day than either FRE or HAF hospices.

Patient-Care Volunteer Hours per Patient Day

An examination of the number of volunteer hours spent in patient-care activities per patient day was undertaken to understand whether the decrease observed according to demonstration status was attributable to the type of activity performed by volunteers: direct patient care or administration. Figures 10.1 and 10.2 present the number of patient-care hours per patient day spent by volunteers by demonstration status and organizational type. Demonstration volunteers spent, on the average, 0.22 hours per patient day in patient-care activities, compared to 0.59 hours in nondemonstration sites. Analysis of variance on twelve-month averages revealed a significant difference according to demonstration status, but no organizational-type effect. A significant interaction ($p = 0.026$) between demonstration status and organizational type, in conjunction with an examination of the pattern of means, suggested that the demonstration effect may have been concentrated among FRE nondemonstration hospices. This pattern is comparable to that observed for total volunteer hours per patient day, indicating that FRE nondemonstration hospices provide significantly more patient-care hours per patient day than their demonstration counterparts.

Further statistical analyses were conducted on these data to determine

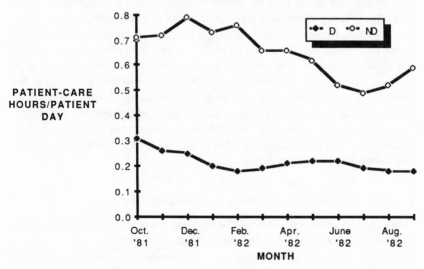

Figure 10.1   Volunteer Patient-Care Hours per Patient Day for Demonstration and Nondemonstration Hospices

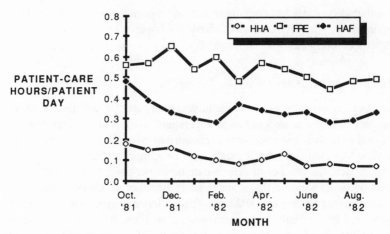

Figure 10.2   Volunteer Patient-Care Hours per Patient Day for Home Health Agency–Based, Hospital-Affiliated, and Freestanding Hospices

whether the passage of time had any effect on the number of volunteer patient-care hours per patient day. Repeated measures analysis of variance results revealed no overall time effect and no differential change as a function of demonstration status. No organizational effect or interaction was observed, suggesting that all three organizational types behaved in a similar manner over time. These statistical analyses contradict the graphical display of data in figures 10.1 and 10.2, which show a slight decrease in volunteer patient-care activity per patient day over the twelve-month period. This decrease in volunteer activity is not statistically significant for either demonstration or organizational groups. In contrast to the significant differential change in total volunteer hours per patient day for demonstration and nondemonstration hospices discussed above, these findings suggest that demonstration and nondemonstration hospices continued to emphasize volunteers' role in patient care despite the availability of reimbursement for these services when delivered by paid staff in demonstration sites. Volunteer patient-care hours per patient day did not decrease significantly over time. Reductions in volunteer time appeared to be restricted to their performance of administrative activities, particularly among nondemonstration FRE organizations.

Changes in Volunteer Use in Relation to Paid Staff Time

When patient census increases and the total number of volunteer hours remains fairly constant, a net decrease in the total number of volunteer hours per patient day results. Since this phenomenon occurred to some extent in both demonstration and nondemonstration hospices, we chose to examine whether the ratio of volunteers to paid staff was related to the decrease in the number of volunteer hours per patient day.

A decreasing ratio would indicate that the hospices were responding to growth in patient census by hiring additional paid staff while failing to recruit additional volunteers. Such a finding might suggest that volunteers were, in fact, being "replaced" by paid staff. The ratio of the number of volunteers to the number of paid staff presented in figure 10.3 indicates a remarkable consistency in demonstration sites over time at a level of approximately one volunteer per paid staff person. In nondemonstration sites, this ratio decreased from a high of 4.8 to a low of 2.4. Statistical analysis substantiated this graphical display, revealing a highly significant demonstration by time effect. Nondemonstration hospices have smaller paid staffs than demonstration sites; even moderate changes in the level of volunteer activity or the number of paid staff could cause these ratios to change greatly. When these same data were examined by organizational type, a similar decrease in the ratio of volunteers to paid staff was observed in FRE hospices. This decrease (fig. 10.4) was confirmed by statistical analysis that indicated highly significant differential rates of change for the three organizational types and an even stronger interaction effect. This pattern suggested that a true organizational effect may exist regardless of demonstration status. To further explore the source of organizational effect, we examined the ratio of volunteers to paid staff in FRE hospices only (fig. 10.5). We found again that nondemonstration FRE hospices behaved quite differently from demonstration FRE hospices over time. The differential change over time for FRE hospices by demonstration status mirrored that which was observed in figure 10.3.

The ratio of volunteer hours to paid staff hours provides another more

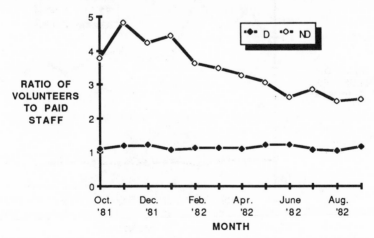

Figure 10.3   Ratio of Volunteers to Paid Staff for Demonstration and Nondemonstration Hospices

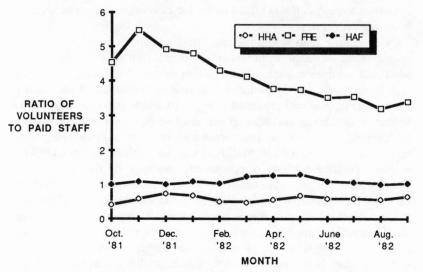

Figure 10.4   Ratio of Volunteers to Paid Staff for Home Health Agency–Based, Hospital-Affiliated, and Freestanding Hospices

sensitive measure of change in the prevalence of volunteers in relation to paid staff. Many hospices employ part-time staff, and the number of hours spent by volunteers is subject to variation. Table 10.5 presents mean values for the initial and final ratios by demonstration status and organizational type. The decrease

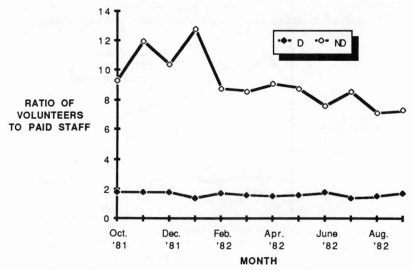

Figure 10.5   Ratio of Volunteers to Paid Staff in Freestanding Hospices (Demonstration and Nondemonstration)

Table 10.5   Average Ratio of Total Volunteer Hours to Total Paid Staff Hours

Measure	Demonstration Status		Total (N = 38)
	Demonstration* (N = 25)	Nondemonstration (N = 13)	
Initial (months 1–3)			
3-month average	.13	.95	.37
standard deviation	.11	1.49	.87
Final (months 10–12)			
3-month average	.11	.48	.22
standard deviation	.09	.74	.42

Measure	Organizational Type			
	HAF (N = 16)	FRE* (N = 12)	HHA (N = 10)	Total (N = 38)
Initial (months 1–3)				
3-month average	.12	.91	.11	.37
standard deviation	.06	1.42	.15	.87
Final (months 10–12)				
3-month average	.10	.52	.08	.22
standard deviation	.06	.72	.12	.42

*Paid staff data are missing from one FRE demonstration hospice.

in the ratio of volunteer time to paid staff time was striking among both nondemonstration and FRE sites. This finding was consistent with changes in the ratio of volunteers to paid staff.

Analysis of variance revealed a significant demonstration effect and organizational effect for the initial measures and for the final measures. Further analysis of these data indicated that the relative contribution of volunteer and paid staff hours changed differentially over time by demonstration status and by organizational type. A significant interaction of demonstration status and organizational type suggested once again that much of the decrease observed was attributable to the nondemonstration FRE hospices.

An examination of volunteer roles once again helped to understand these findings. The ratio of volunteer patient-care hours to direct-care paid staff hours compared the time volunteers actually spent with patients to all hours worked by all paid staff whose primary function was patient care. Although useful for comparison purposes, this ratio does not give an absolute measure of the hours spent by paid staff in actual patient care. Table 10.6 presents mean values for the ratio of volunteer patient-care hours to total direct-care paid staff hours. Significant differences in initial measures were observed for demonstration status and organizational type. Comparing the final measures revealed no significant difference by either demonstration status or organizational type, suggesting that these groups may have begun to approach similar levels of direct-care volunteer activity in relation to their direct-care paid staff time. We exam-

Table 10.6   Average Ratio of Total Volunteer Patient-Care Hours to Patient-Care Paid Staff Hours

| Measure | Demonstration Status | | Total |
	Demonstration* (N = 25)	Nondemonstration (N = 13)	(N = 38)
Initial (months 1–3)			
3-month average	.07	.69	.23
standard deviation	.05	1.25	.66
Final (months 10–12)			
3-month average	.08	.18	.11
standard deviation	.18	.45	.27

| Measure | Organizational Type | | | |
	HAF (N = 16)	FRE* (N = 12)	HHA (N = 10)	Total (N = 38)
Initial (months 1–3)				
3-month average	.09	.64	.05	.23
standard deviation	.04	1.18	.04	.66
Final (months 10–12)				
3-month average	.13	.16	.03	.11
standard deviation	.16	.48	.13	.27

*Paid staff data are missing from one FRE demonstration hospice.

ined this proposition more carefully by testing for differences in the variation between hospices of the same type. The variability suggested, and statistical analyses confirmed, that nondemonstration FRE hospices were behaving differently. The ratio of volunteer patient-care hours to direct-care paid staff hours was stable in demonstration sites, but sharply decreased among nondemonstration and FRE sites.

We also examined the ratio of volunteer patient-care hours to direct-care paid staff patient-care hours over time. Statistical analysis revealed a significant change over time for all sites. Considered in light of the values presented in table 10.4, these results suggest that the time effect was attributable to nondemonstration and FRE hospices, which showed a significant decrease in the ratio of volunteer patient-care time to direct-care paid staff time. These sites appeared to be responding to increases in patient census by hiring both administrative and direct-care staff.

Volunteer use in relation to paid staff time remained very stable in demonstration sites, while a pronounced change was observed in nondemonstration FRE sites throughout the NHS. In spite of the absence of Medicare revenues, these nondemonstration (ND) hospices, which began as volunteer-dominated organizations, appeared to substitute paid staff for volunteer staff. Although the decreases observed over time were significant, the contribution made by volunteers in FRE and ND hospices was still two to three times greater than that observed in their non-FRE and demonstration (D) counterparts.

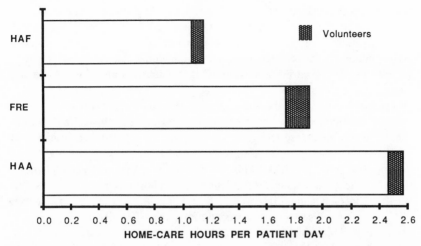

Figure 10.6   Average Home-Care Hours by Volunteers and Paid Staff in Demonstration Sites

The data gathered for the National Hospice Study also made it possible to compare the time volunteers spent making home visits with the hours actually spent by paid staff and reimbursed by Medicare. These data were only available for NHS demonstration hospices and may not be representative of other hospices. As can be seen in figure 10.6, HHA hospices delivered over 2.5 hours of home care per patient day, which is over twice the level reported for HAF hospices. Volunteers accounted for 4.3 percent and 7.4 percent of these home-care hours in HHA and HAF hospices, respectively, whereas volunteers in FRE hospices delivered 9 percent of the home-care hours per patient day.

The Future of the Hospice Volunteer

If the trends observed in NHS hospices are generalizable, the activities of the hospice volunteer may be shifting toward increased time with patients and away from clerical and administrative tasks. This shift may be a response to the hospices' attempts to meet the multiplicity of patients' needs in a cost-effective manner. We do not have specific data on whether volunteer time on the hospice board of directors and involvement in other community activities has decreased, but anecdotal evidence from FRE hospices suggests that hospice boards are becoming more traditional in their composition (i.e., attorneys, physicians, executives).

While the increased use of voluntary labor for patient care may be considered a positive outcome for hospices, this use of volunteers is not without cost to the hospice. There are costs associated with the more intensive recruitment, screening, training, and supervision that may be required to administer this voluntary labor force. This greater investment by hospices in their volunteer programs may lead to new demands on the volunteers themselves. Could demands such as a required caseload, attendance at staff meetings, and maintenance of patient progress notes impede volunteer recruitment efforts or produce high volunteer turnover? On the other hand, could the extensive training, supervision, and experience be so good that volunteers are "lost" to paying jobs?

The NHS experience and subsequent observations suggest that the role of the hospice volunteer may become better defined and more formalized. Volunteers as a resource were recognized by Congress in 1982 when it mandated Medicare coverage of hospice services as part of the Tax Equity and Fiscal Responsibility Act (TEFRA). This legislation and the regulations implementing it include volunteers under the definition of a hospice employee and stipulate that a hospice maintain records on the use of volunteers and the cost savings and expansion of services achieved through their use. Each hospice must document and maintain a level of volunteer activity that, at a minimum, equals 5 percent of the total patient-care hours of all paid staff. NHS findings indicate that the maintenance of this level of volunteer activity is both feasible and reasonable, at least in the hospices studied. To achieve cost savings and expansion of services, however, may require hospices to make new demands of their volunteers. While productivity may not have been critical in the past, it may take on added significance for hospice volunteers under TEFRA. Will TEFRA lead to the "professional hospice volunteer"? The experience of hospice volunteers under this new legislation should be examined in future research to determine the effect of regulations on volunteerism in the health-care industry.

While the TEFRA volunteer requirement was intended to help assure that hospice care retains those qualities that made it a unique and responsive service, the formalization of the role of the hospice volunteer could have unintended results. Since other sectors of the health-care system have experienced an expansion in professional liability, hospices (and potentially volunteers themselves) may more frequently become targets of litigation (Laliberte and Mor 1985). We saw that many hospice volunteers were either active or retired health-care professionals. These individuals may not wish to subject themselves to potential liability without compensation. If hospices wish to recruit such individuals into their volunteer programs, one feature that could attract many health-care and other professionals is liability insurance to cover their hospice activities. The issue of liability for volunteer activities is one that should be addressed by hospice governing boards.

Conclusion

The initiative and energy of hospice volunteers have helped identify the need and gain public support for a new concept in health care. This grass-roots effort gained momentum and achieved legitimacy prior to the HCFA demonstration and NHS. Subsequent legislation provided for the inclusion of hospice care as a service reimbursed by many health insurance carriers, including Medicare.

As an integral part of the hospice movement, volunteers were the focus of many questions posed by the NHS. We found that they were typical of human service volunteers in general—white, female, middle-aged, and well educated. Their activities ranged from the provision of skilled care (e.g., nursing) to companionship, emotional counseling, and the meeting of concrete needs such as transportation. No other provider group seems better equipped to meet the multiplicity of needs of dying patients and their families.

There appeared to be a sufficient pool of volunteers in all settings. We saw that nondemonstration hospices, particularly those freestanding sites that were not affiliated with a hospital or home health agency, utilized volunteers to a greater degree than other sites. As we expected, the level of volunteers' involvement did decrease over time in demonstration sites. We were surprised to discover that this decrease did not reflect a decrease in the level of patient care provided by volunteers but, rather, indicated less involvement in administrative activities. This finding suggested that volunteer programs in demonstration sites were expanding with their increasing patient census and that any reductions in the total hours per patient day should be attributed either to decreases in volunteer administrative time or reallocations of volunteers from administrative to patient-care activities.

The ratio of volunteers to paid staff was remarkably stable at a level of approximately 1.0 in demonstration sites compared to the decreases observed in nondemonstration sites. Nondemonstration FRE hospices had the highest ratio of volunteers to paid staff but showed the most rapid decreases in this ratio over time. This indicated that additional paid staff were being hired. As these hospices continue to grow we may see this decrease continue until the organizations reach the relatively stable levels of volunteer involvement observed in demonstration sites.

An examination of the ratio of volunteer hours to paid staff hours produced similar results. Nondemonstration FRE sites experienced a higher ratio and a more rapid decrease in this ratio over time. When this ratio of volunteer hours to paid staff hours was examined for only patient-care time, the decreases observed over time were also attributable to nondemonstration FRE hospices, which have responded to increases in patient census by hiring both administrative and direct-care staff. Demonstration sites, however, appeared to have increased the number of hours spent by paid administrative staff as well as the relative level of volunteer patient-care time.

Regardless of the availability of reimbursement, volunteers continue to be a valuable resource for hospices, particularly inpatient-care activities. Volunteers carry out a wide variety of functions, including direct care, but also staff support, fund-raising, and public relations. They comprise a unique human resource for hospice organizations as representatives of the community who make a gift of their time, sensitivity, and concern to patients and families attempting to cope with terminal illness and bereavement. Their services are not free, however; agency resources are expended in their recruitment, screening, training, support, and supervision. Unlike paid staff, volunteers do not present substantial fixed costs that must be carried regardless of radical shifts in patient census. Once trained, they represent a potential resource pool to be drawn upon for relatively short-term involvement with patients until their deaths.

11

Organizational Growth and Change among Hospices

LINDA LALIBERTE
AND VINCENT MOR

The hospice movement in the United States has been characterized as a social phenomenon (Stoddard 1978). Its philosophy has been based on the idealistic and zealous commitment of its leaders and volunteers. Central to the hospice movement has been its concern for the psychological and spiritual well-being of both the person facing death and his or her family. In large part, the movement arose as an expression of the belief that the dying person needs emotional comfort as well as competent professional care. The hospice philosophy has from the start emphasized the active role of family members and other supportive individuals and envisioned home care as a viable alternative to the traditional institutional setting. Given the deficiency of financial resources, it was not surprising that early hospices were staffed primarily by volunteers—members of religious groups, health-care professionals, and members of the general public. These volunteers not only provided services to patients and their families but also promoted the hospice to others in the community, thereby advancing the movement.

In the course of providing services to growing numbers of terminally ill patients, this social movement evolved into a system of care. Various organizations were spawned to provide the patterns of care advocated. The first were those voluntary associations whose sole purpose was to implement the hospice philosophy. However, because the movement was broad based, staff in established health-care organizations soon developed specialty units to serve hospice patients. Although hospices have assumed diverse organizational structures, three main classifications of hospice providers have emerged: the original freestanding organizations (FRE) established through the efforts of grass-roots volunteer groups and providing only hospice care with or without inpatient beds, hospital-affiliated hospices (HAF), and home health agency–based hospices (HHA).

Organizations have been described as the social mechanism used to coordinate the activities of a large number of people toward a common goal (Kimberly and Miles 1980). In studying the life cycle of an organization, Downs (1966) notes that the early stage is the most precarious; the organization strives for autonomy by generating external support in the form of resources and a recognized need for its service or product. Growth follows this initial stage, and with growth comes the rigidity associated with bureaucracy (Downs 1966). Bureaucratization was characterized by Weber (1947) as the embodiment of a rationality that relies on structural hierarchy, rules (formalization), and specialization.

The themes advanced by bureaucratization, formalization, and specialization appear to be antithetical to the notion of volunteerism espoused by the hospice movement. Thus the question arises: Can hospices obtain the resources and control necessary for their survival as organizations and at the same time preserve those unique features that have contributed to their effectiveness and success? One answer may lie in the integration of hospices into the traditional health-care system. While the benefits to the hospice could be substantial—access to third-party reimbursement, increased status in the medical community—integration may also present problems. In a study of forty-eight hospice programs in a Midwest community, Paradis (1984) examined this concept of integration. She found that the achievement of integration was often accompanied by increased fragmentation among hospice providers. Competition with traditional providers also developed. Although integrated and nonintegrated hospices showed no significant differences in the types of services provided, integrated hospices placed greater emphasis on hiring paid staff rather than using volunteers (Paradis 1984).

Although little documentation is available on the relative growth of health organizations, the ambulatory-care literature indicates that hospital programs often begin larger and grow faster because of their large resource base. Paradis (1984) found that size was positively related to integration and indicated that many integrated programs were institutionally affiliated. This relationship suggests that hospices that developed within existing organizations (i.e., HAF and HHA hospices) may demonstrate different rates of growth than FRE hospices. We hypothesized that the revenues available to hospices under the demonstration would result in more rapid growth than that observed in nondemonstration hospices.

This chapter describes the changes experienced by NHS hospices. Since the presence of Medicare demonstration funding may have facilitated expansion at a more rapid rate than would otherwise be expected by guaranteeing full reimbursement for hospice costs, the NHS examined growth experienced related to the availability of Medicare reimbursement. The evaluation design made it possible to compare these experiences to those of hospices without guaranteed reimbursement and also to examine the relationship of hospice organizational type to these same factors associated with growth, regardless of the availability of reimbursement.

Method of Analysis

Characteristics of patients and staff in demonstration and nondemonstration hospices were examined at three-month intervals (i.e., quarterly) over a one-year period. The number of observations was the number of hospices—forty. With such a small number of cases, differences over time had to be very large in order to be statistically significant. It was decided to plot values and examine the graphic data for trends. Analysis of variance was used to examine average differences as a result of demonstration status or hospice organizational type, and repeated measures analysis of variance was used to detect differential changes over time.

Data Sources

Hospice Patient Intake and Discharge Data.   NHS data collectors completed intake and discharge forms on all hospice admissions from 8/1/81 through 9/30/82 in demonstration sites and between 8/1/81 and 9/15/82 in nondemonstration hospices. The intake form included demographic, diagnostic, and functional descriptors of patients admitted to hospices. The discharge form reported date of discharge, number of inpatient days spent in the hospice, and the site of the patient's death.

Staff Data.   Each site (except one FRE demonstration hospice) submitted a report of the number of staff employed, the number who resigned, and the number of new staff hired for each of the eight quarters of the demonstration period (for demonstration sites) or for the NHS data-collection period (for nondemonstration sites). These reports were the source of data on the number of paid staff employed by each hospice. Staff time sheets were also completed on a randomly selected weekday each month.

Volunteer Data.   NHS data collectors at each participating site submitted monthly summaries of reported volunteer activity for the NHS data-collection period. The items reported include number of volunteers and the hours they spent in patient care and/or administrative activities.

Sample

The comparison samples being used in this analysis were the HCFA demonstration hospices and the fourteen nondemonstration hospices selected by the evaluator to participate in the NHS. The demonstration sites were twenty-seven in number for this analysis. They were distributed by organizational structure as follows: ten were affiliated with hospitals (HAF), eight with home health agencies (HHA), and nine were freestanding (FRE) organizations with no institutional affiliation. The fourteen nondemonstration sites selected by Brown as comparison sites represented a similar distribution—eight were HAF, two were HHA, and four were FRE.

Although the nondemonstration sites were selected to comprise a group of hospices similar to the HCFA demonstration sites, the two groups were not identical. In selecting the demonstration sites from among the 233 applicant organizations, HCFA considered the comprehensiveness of the hospice intervention, the soundness and thoroughness of the service plan in the proposal, and whether the hospice was operational. By definition, then, demonstration sites had been operational at least one year, and the demonstration was in its tenth month by the time NHS data collection began. In addition, the reporting requirements necessitated by the demonstration may have contributed to the inclusion of hospices at higher levels of organizational development.

Examining the Rates of Change over Time

The analyses reported in this chapter compared the rates of change in case mix, number of staff, and volunteer activity in demonstration and nondemonstration hospices. The data were aggregated by quarter, plotted, and examined for trends to determine whether hospices changed differentially over time with respect to demonstration status or organizational type. Analysis of variance was then used to determine whether differences in averages over the quarters being examined were statistically significant. Because the number of cases was only forty-one and any differences would have to be very large to be significant, a probability value of .10 was accepted as an indicator of significance.

Dependent Variables

Two classes of dependent variables were used in this analysis—aggregated patient variables and staff variables. Patient variables included the number of admissions, age distribution, diagnosis, living arrangement, functional status, Medicare status, length of stay, and total number of days in the hospice for each quarter's admission cohort. Staff variables included the number of paid staff employed each quarter and the ratio of volunteers to paid staff. A description of the variables and their hypothesized relationship to demonstration status and organizational structure follows:

- *Number of admissions and total hospice days* provide measures of the volume of patients served by NHS hospices. An increase in the number of admissions per quarter would be consistent with growth of the hospice. With the availability of Medicare reimbursement, demonstration sites were expected to grow faster than nondemonstration hospices.

- *Age distribution, diagnosis, and number of Medicare patients* are measures used to analyze case mix, that is, the profile of the group of patients admitted to hospices. An increase in the age distribution and number of patients with a primary diagnosis other than cancer would be consistent with an increase in the number of Medicare patients being served. Demonstration hospices may focus on Medicare patients to maximize reimbursement under the demonstration.

- *Functional status and length of stay* are also measures used to analyze case mix. Functional status is a measure constructed from the assessment of the patient's abilities to perform activities of daily living. This assessment was modeled on the Katz et al. (1963) ADL Index. A decrease in the patient's functional status at admission and a shorter length of stay would indicate that more dependent patients are entering the hospice in the very last stages of their illness. This finding could also be related to increased utilization of inpatient resources.

- *Patient living arrangement and PCP support* provide measures of the level of support available at home. Patients who live alone or do not live with their PCPs may rely more on hospice service resources. PCP support is defined as low when there is no PCP. Other gross indicators of lower levels of PCP support are a PCP who does not live with the patient, a PCP who is employed, or a PCP who is over seventy-five years of age. These are used as indicators based on the assumption that a PCP who works or does not live with the patient is less available to provide for the patient. Use of the PCP age as an indicator is based upon the decline in functional status that is known to occur as part of the aging process. The absence of strong informal support at home can be assumed to place a greater demand on the hospice to provide intensive home services or inpatient care.

- *Number of staff* employed each quarter provides a measure of the growth experienced by the hospice. An increase in the volume of patients may be accompanied by an increase in the number of direct-care staff. The reporting requirements imposed by the HCFA demonstration may be related to increases in the number of administrative staff.

- *Ratio of volunteers to paid staff* is an indicator of the level of volunteer involvement. A decrease in the ratio may be a by-product of rapid growth and increased bureaucratization experienced by some organizations. This measure indicates whether the availability of reimbursement could pose a threat to the unique resource of volunteers.

Results

The Impact of Reimbursement on the Volume and Case Mix of Patients

Experience in other sectors of the health-care industry led us to hypothesize that Medicare reimbursement would accelerate growth in demonstration hospices beyond that seen in nondemonstration hospices and that Medicare patients would represent a greater proportion of the case mix over time. We examined the number of admissions, total hospice days, and the proportion of Medicare patients per quarter in demonstration and nondemonstration hospices.

Volume of Hospice Patients

Figure 11.1 presents the number of admissions per quarter for the NHS data-collection period (year 2 of the HCFA demonstration). As can be seen, demonstration sites served more patients than nondemonstration hospices at the outset and continued to do so throughout the study. The number of admissions in demonstration hospices showed a steady increase, while admissions at nondemonstration sites showed a slight decrease. Analysis of variance on the average number of admissions per site over the four quarters revealed a significant demonstration effect ($p < .01$). Repeated measures analysis of variance revealed no significant change in the number of admissions across all sites as a function of time; however, a significant ($p = .026$) differential change in the number of admissions per quarter was observed as a function of demonstration

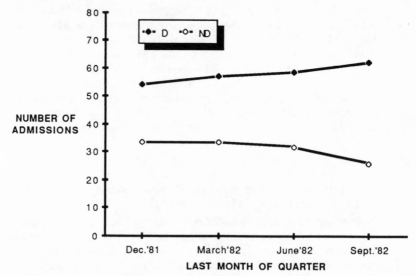

Figure 11.1   Number of Admissions per Quarter at Demonstration and Nondemonstration Hospices

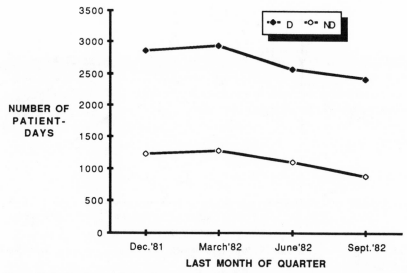

Figure 11.2   Number of Patient Days per Quarter at Demonstration and Nondemonstration Hospices

status. A similar pattern was found for the total number of hospice days presented in figure 11.2. Demonstration hospices provided an average of 2,698 days of hospice care per quarter compared to 1,214 days in nondemonstration sites. Analysis of variance on these averages confirmed that the difference in the number of hospice patient days utilized by the two groups was significant ($p < .025$). Contrary to the finding regarding number of admissions, repeated measures analysis of variance on these data revealed a significant ($p = .001$) overall time effect but no differential change as a function of demonstration status. These conflicting results suggested that the observed time effects may be due to quarterly fluctuations in the data rather than being representative of a consistent trend.

Case Mix of Hospice Patients

Demonstration hospices served more patients than nondemonstration sites. In order to better understand the impact of reimbursement on these observed differences, the proportion of Medicare patients served over four quarters was examined (fig. 11.3). An average of 71.9 percent of all patients admitted to demonstration hospices were Medicare recipients, compared to 62.6 percent of nondemonstration hospice patients. This difference was indicative of significance at $p < .10$. The data in figure 11.3 suggested that demonstration hospices were attracting those Medicare recipients seeking hospice services. The proportion of Medicare patients served by nondemonstration hospices decreased

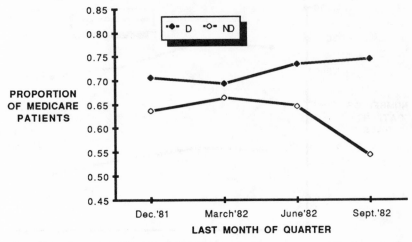

Figure 11.3   Proportion of Medicare Patients Admitted to Demonstration and Nondemonstration Hospices

sharply during the last six months of the data-collection period, while increasing numbers of Medicare patients were being admitted to demonstration hospices. Results of a repeated measures analysis of variance on these data confirmed the presence of a significant differential change ($p = .028$) as a function of demonstration status, but no overall time effect was observed.

This shift in the proportion of Medicare patients at demonstration hospices was also reflected in the age distribution of patients at these sites. Figure 11.4 shows that a greater percentage of patients serviced in demonstration hospices were over sixty-five years of age—65 percent compared to 59 percent in non-demonstration hospices. Averaged over the four quarters, this difference in age distribution was not significant. Repeated measures analysis of variance was indicative of significance ($p < .081$) and suggested that, over time, demonstration hospices began to serve a greater proportion of patients over sixty-five years of age.

An examination of other case-mix descriptors over time revealed that an increasing proportion of patients was served by both hospice groups for less than seven days. No other trends were observed. The average values for the measures presented in table 11.1 suggest that the two groups of hospices were quite similar. A greater proportion of nondemonstration patients appeared to be short-stay patients. This may be a function of the disproportionate number of nondemonstration patients served at HAF hospices, however. Slightly more patients in nondemonstration sites also had weaker PCP support than patients in demonstration sites. This latter finding may be related to the requirement that demonstration participants have a PCP and to the larger number of HAF non-demonstration hospices. As will be seen in the next section, the availability of

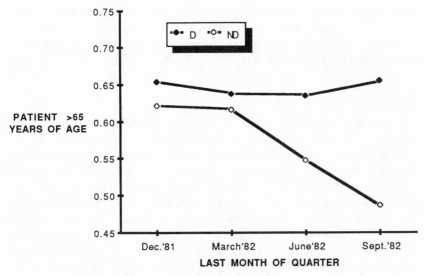

Figure 11.4   Proportion of Patients over Sixty-Five Years of Age at Demonstration and Non-demonstration Hospices

inpatient beds in HAF hospices may have attracted those patients with weaker levels of support at home.

The Relationship of Hospice Organizational Type to the Volume and Case Mix of Patients

We saw that the availability of reimbursement led to more rapid expansion among demonstration hospices and a case mix that shifted toward a greater

Table 11.1   Average Case-Mix Measures over Last Four Quarters of the National Hospice Study

	Demonstration ($\bar{x}$)	Nondemonstration ($\bar{x}$)	Significance
Proportion of patients with length of stay less than 7 days	.19	.26	$p < .10$
Mean functional status score*	8.42	7.91	NS
Proportion of patients living alone	.13	.19	NS
Proportion of patients with weak PCP support	.24	.36	NS
Proportion of patients with diagnosis other than cancer	.11	.12	NS

*Seven activities of daily living reported on each patient's intake form were assigned the following values: 1 = can do alone, 2 = can do with assistance, 3 = unable to do alone. These values were summed for the seven activities to give a functional status score for each patient. A mean functional status score was calculated for each site.

NS = Not Significant.

proportion of Medicare patients. In view of the different organizational origins of the hospices in our sample, we examined the same variables across the three organizational types to determine whether relationships existed regardless of the availability of reimbursement.

Volume of Hospice Patients

The number of admissions per quarter for each organizational type are present-ed in figure 11.5. As can be seen, FRE and HHA hospices served more patients than HAF hospices throughout the study. Analysis of variance on the averages for the four quarters confirmed an organizational effect approaching signifi-cance ($p < .10$). While FRE hospices showed a steady growth in the number of patients served, HAF and HHA hospices revealed only quarterly fluctuations. Repeated measures analysis of variance on these data revealed no significant trends over time. The number of patient days (fig. 11.6) reflected the numbers of admissions. HHA hospices served an average of 3,093 patient days per quarter as compared to 2,779 patient days for FRE patients and 1,269 for HAF patients. Differences in the average number of days patients spent in the hospice were significant at $p < .025$. Although repeated measures analysis of variance revealed an overall time effect ($p = .001$), the decrease observed in the number of patient days may be an artifact due to increasing numbers of patients in the quarterly admission cohorts who were not discharged by the end of the study or for whom discharge data were not available.

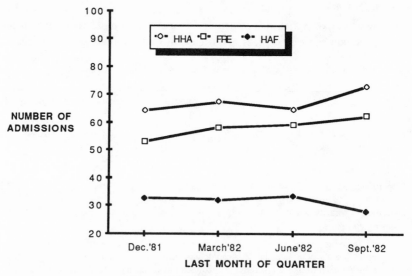

Figure 11.5   Number of Admissions per Quarter at Hospital-Affiliated, Home Health Agency–Based, and Freestanding Hospices

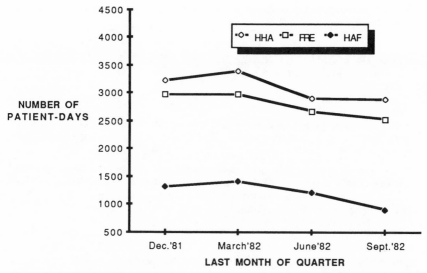

Figure 11.6   Number of Patient Days per Quarter at Hospital-Affiliated, Home Health Agency–
Based, and Freestanding Hospices

Case Mix of Hospice Patients

We observed that demonstration hospices began to serve a greater proportion of
Medicare beneficiaries, while nondemonstration hospices served a smaller
proportion. We saw no such shift related to the hospices' organizational structure. Freestanding hospices served fewer Medicare patients than hospital-affiliated hospices, and there were no changes in the proportion of Medicare patients
served over time. There were no significant differences in the averages among
the three groups, nor was there a significant time effect related to organizational
type. The lower proportion of Medicare patients in FRE sites was consistent
with the lower percentage of patients over the age of sixty-five served in these
sites.

We examined factors related to the type of patient being served by these three
groups of hospices. Over the four quarters being studied, the proportion of
short-stay patients increased in all three organizational types. Since less than 10
percent of hospice patients are discharged alive, this increase in the proportion
of short-stay patients meant that more patients were being admitted to hospices
during the week preceding their death. As hospice care was gaining momentum
during the years of the HCFA demonstration, there may have been less debate
or reluctance among traditional providers of care to refer these end-stage terminal patients to the hospice. Whether this trend will continue remains to be seen.
As can be seen in table 11.2, 25 percent of HAF patients were served by the
hospice for seven days or less. The average over four quarters was significantly

Table 11.2   Average Case-Mix Measures over Last Four Quarters of the National
Hospice Study

	HAF ($\bar{x}$)	HHA ($\bar{x}$)	FRE ($\bar{x}$)	Significance
Proportion of patients with length of stay less than 7 days	.26	.17	.18	$p < .10$
Mean functional status score*	8.64	8.32	7.70	NS
Proportion of patients living alone	.21	.11	.10	$p < .025$
Proportion of patients with weak PCP support	.36	.23	.23	NS
Proportion of patients with diagnosis other than cancer	.15	.14	.06	$p < .10$

*Seven activities of daily living reported on each patient's intake form were assigned the following values: 1 = can do alone, 2 = can do with assistance, 3 = unable to do alone. These values were summed for the seven activities to give a functional status score for each patient. A mean functional status score was calculated for each site.
NS = Not Significant.

different ($p < .10$) from both FRE hospices (18 percent) and HHA hospices (17.7 percent). These data also suggest that FRE hospices served primarily cancer patients who were less functionally impaired and did not live alone. HHA hospices served slightly more noncancer patients, but otherwise resembled the FRE hospices. HAF hospices served approximately the same proportion of noncancer patients as did HHA hospices. The similarity ends there. Patients in HAF hospices were more functionally impaired, had weaker PCP support, and were more likely to live alone. This pattern was constant over all quarters examined, suggesting that patient selection and referral patterns to the three types of hospices, though different, were consistent.

The Impact of Reimbursement on the Staffing of Hospices

We hypothesized that Medicare reimbursement would accelerate growth in demonstration hospices, and we saw that the number of admissions increased more rapidly in these sites than in their nondemonstration counterparts. A corollary to this hypothesis was the assumption that changes in patient census would be accompanied by changes in the level and distribution of staffing.

As can be seen in figure 11.7, demonstration hospices employed more staff and appeared to be hiring additional staff to care for their growing patient census. The growth observed in the level of staff at nondemonstration hospices was less pronounced, suggesting that it occurred as part of their normal organizational development. Analysis of variance on the means for the four quarters indicated a difference approaching significance as a result of demonstration status ($p < .10$). No significant time effect was obtained in repeated measures analysis of variance, indicating the absence of an overall trend as well as a differential rate of change for the two groups.

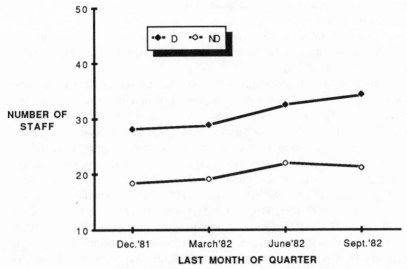

Figure 11.7   Number of Staff per Quarter at Demonstration and Nondemonstration Hospices

The literature on organizational development indicates that increased bureaucratization may accompany growth. We hypothesized that the availability of reimbursement and the rapid growth associated with it would lead to an increased proportion of administrative staff in demonstration hospices. As can be seen in figure 11.8, we found that the proportion of administrative staff decreased slightly in demonstration and nondemonstration hospices, indicating that many of the additional staff being hired were direct-care staff. Analysis of

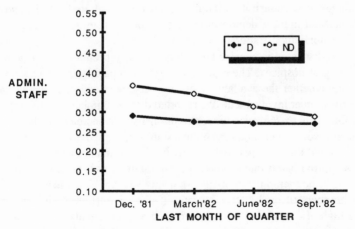

Figure 11.8   Proportion of Administrative Staff per Quarter at Demonstration and Nondemonstration Hospices

variance on the means for the four quarters indicated no significant difference as a result of demonstration status. Repeated measures analysis of variance revealed a significant ($p = .053$) overall time effect but no differential changes in the proportion of administrative staff employed over the four quarters as a result of demonstration status.

Changes in the number of staff were occurring, but it was not clear how time was being allocated. We examined the proportion of administrative time spent by all hospice staff and by nurses alone (Mor et al. 1985). Administrative time was classified as general (nonpatient related) and patient related (e.g., case management, care planning, interdisciplinary team meetings). We found that staff in demonstration hospices spent a significantly greater proportion of their time performing both types of administrative activities. Once again we examined quarterly averages in demonstration and nondemonstration hospices to detect a change over time. Repeated measures analysis of variance indicated no significant differential change in the proportion of administrative time spent by all hospice staff or by nurses alone. Since demonstration hospices were guaranteed reimbursement, staff presumably could afford to spend more time serving this administrative function.

Advocates of hospice care have argued that the provision of home services to terminally ill patients requires more time than is normally allocated for such home visits. Since the Medicare limits on reimbursement for nursing and other home visits were eliminated under the demonstration, hospice staff had a certain degree of flexibility to spend whatever time was necessary in caring for their patients. Data on over five thousand reported patient visits conducted over twelve months were examined to determine the intensity of the hospice home visit (Mor et al. 1985). The average duration of a hospice nursing visit (travel plus visit time) was about 1.5 hours. There was a difference in the length of visit as a function of demonstration status, but it was concentrated in HHA and FRE hospices. Staff in these demonstration sites reported significantly longer visits than their nondemonstration counterparts.

As was discussed in chapter 10, volunteers have been a unique resource in the staffing of hospices. The ratio of volunteers to paid staff was examined to determine whether the availability of reimbursement caused a change in the level of volunteer involvement. We reported that the number of staff employed by hospices increased over time. A commensurate increase in the level of volunteer involvement should result in a stable ratio of volunteers to paid staff. We found that this ratio was remarkably consistent in demonstration sites at a level of approximately one volunteer per paid staff person. More variability was observed in nondemonstration sites, but this was largely influenced by their lower numbers of paid staff. The ratio at nondemonstration sites decreased from a high of 4.8 to a low of 2.4. Repeated measures analysis of variance on these ratios revealed no significant overall time effect but a highly significant ($p < .001$) time by demonstration status interaction effect.

The Effect of Organizational Structure on Hospice Staffing Level

We observed that reimbursement accelerated growth in patient census, in the number of staff employed in demonstration hospices, and in the proportion of time spent by staff in administrative activities. We examined staffing levels to determine whether there was any relationship to organizational structure, regardless of the availability of reimbursement.

The staff data presented in figure 11.9 correspond to the admission data presented in figure 11.4. HHA and FRE sites showed staff growth, while HAF sites maintained a stable level. However, repeated measures analysis of variance did not indicate a significant differential change over time. Analysis of variance on the means over four quarters indicated a significant difference ($p < .10$) in staffing levels as a result of organizational type. HAF hospices employed an average of 21.3 staff, compared to 24.3 for FRE sites and 39.2 for HHA sites.

The proportion of administrative staff in FRE hospices was twice that observed in either HHA or HAF sites, as can be seen in figure 11.10, suggesting that the agency-based hospices may rely upon their affiliates for administrative support. Analysis of variance confirms a highly significant difference at $p < .005$ as a result of organizational type. An average of 53.4 percent of staff employed in FRE hospices were administrative as compared to 19 percent in HAF and HHA sites. Repeated measures analysis of variance on these data revealed a significant trend toward a decrease in the percentage of admin-

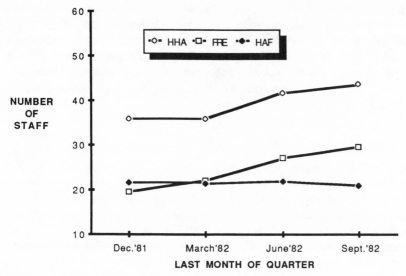

Figure 11.9   Number of Staff per Quarter at Hospital-Affiliated, Home Health Agency–Based, and Freestanding Hospices

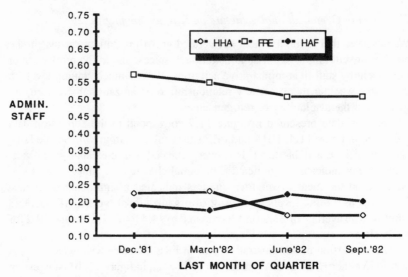

Figure 11.10   Proportion of Administrative Staff at Hospital-Affiliated, Home Health Agency–Based, and Freestanding Hospices

istrative support at all sites, but no significant differential change related to organizational type.

The ratio of volunteers to paid staff was examined by organizational type. The decrease observed in the ratio at FRE sites was similar to what was seen in nondemonstration sites, suggesting that the trend observed in nondemonstration data may be largely due to the FRE sites with large numbers of volunteers and very few paid staff. Repeated measures analysis of variance confirmed a significant ($p = .004$) differential rate of change as a result of organizational type and a significant ($p < .001$) interaction effect, suggesting that the organizational effect may be concentrated more among the nondemonstration hospices.

Summary

In this examination of factors related to the changes experienced by hospice organizations, we saw that the availability of reimbursement in demonstration sites stimulated growth in the number of patients admitted to hospices. This growth was most pronounced among FRE sites. Demonstration sites served a greater proportion of Medicare beneficiaries than did nondemonstration hospices. There were no significant differences in the proportion of Medicare patients across the three organizational types.

An examination of case-mix descriptors revealed that an increasing proportion of short-stay patients were being served at all hospices, regardless of demonstration status or organizational type. On the average, 25 percent of HAF patients were served by the hospice for seven days or less, compared to 18 percent of FRE patients and 17 percent of HHA patients. Patients in HAF hospices were more functionally impaired, had weaker PCP support, and were more likely to live alone. The availability of an inpatient unit in HAF hospices may attract a more vulnerable group of patients. The increasing proportion of short-stay patients may have been a by-product of the integration of hospice care into the traditional health-care system. Members of the medical community who had never referred patients to such a program were, perhaps, less reluctant to refer patients who were already in the last days of their lives.

Growth in patient census at demonstration sites was accompanied by an increase in the number of staff at these sites. Although demonstration hospices employed significantly more staff than nondemonstration sites, the rate of growth in staff size was not significantly different for the two groups. Staff growth did appear to be more concentrated among FRE and HHA hospices. The proportion of administrative staff showed a slight but steady decrease across all sites, suggesting that increased bureaucratization may not be a concomitant effect of rapid growth. FRE hospices employed a significantly higher proportion of administrative staff, but they also used more volunteers.

The ratio of volunteers to paid staff was remarkably stable in demonstration sites at a level of approximately one volunteer per paid staff person, suggesting that the availability of reimbursement did not threaten this resource. While a decrease in the ratio was observed in nondemonstration hospices, it was concentrated among those FRE organizations that were only minimally staffed by paid personnel and relied upon volunteers for most services.

We must be cautious in interpreting and extrapolating from these findings. Conditions of participation in the demonstration project were very different from what will take place as a result of TEFRA. Our sample of hospices was not random. They were selected in part because of the soundness and size of their programs. We must keep this caveat in mind when interpreting these findings. The Medicare hospice benefit may result in larger hospices that are more dependent on paid staff and that rely on Medicare for their revenue.

Differences in the mix of patients served suggest that if HAF hospices continue to admit patients with weak informal support, they may have difficulty keeping patients at home and meeting TEFRA's 20 percent maximum on inpatient days. An increase in the percentage of short-stay patients occurred across all sites; for short-length-of-stay patients, only minimal cost savings may accrue vis-à-vis conventional care. Given the proposed TEFRA rate structure, an increase in the number of short-stay patients could mean that a disproportionate number of patient days would require intensive home services, thus driving up the costs per day at home. Finally, in the short run, reimbursement need not result in diminished volunteer involvement. Provisions in the TEFRA regulations for maintenance of volunteer effort as a proportion of all staff patient-care time are reasonable and could be met by almost all participating NHS hospices.

12

Public Policy and the Hospice Movement

DAVID S. GREER,
VINCENT MOR,
AND ROBERT KASTENBAUM

What is the driving purpose behind the hospice movement in the United States? Two very different answers suggest themselves: "Improve the quality of life for terminally ill people and their families" and "Hold costs down." It is the humanistic motive that is largely responsible for the introduction of the hospice concept and its first realizations in practice. The fiscal motive, however, has been a prime factor in the willingness of the federal government and the health insurance industry to experiment with Medicare reimbursement for hospice services—as well as to support evaluation efforts such as the study reported in this book.

One could hardly have devised a more promising plot for dramatic conflict. Is it really possible that humanitarian impulse and fiscal conservatism can achieve synergy? Or must the hospice movement eventually fall victim to policy analysts whose concerns seldom stray from financial considerations? The opportunity for long-term success of the hospice movement within the economic and ideologic marketplace would seem to require an unusually fortuitous set of circumstances. Of key significance would be (1) the ability of hospices to perform in accordance with their own goals and objectives, (2) the actual achievement of these goals and objectives in patient-family care, and (3) evidence that the hospice alternative represents an appreciable cost savings over traditional care. This scenario would presumably result in the continued growth and support of hospice programs. However, it is a scenario vulnerable to a myriad of external forces. Increased resistance of physicians to making hospice referrals, a decrease in the pool of volunteers, or a new set of statistical assumptions regarding the reimbursement formulas—any of these situations, and many more, could upset the precarious balance between the humanitarian and fiscal policy impulse. The problems themselves might arise from other sources than hospice operation per se; for example, an increasing number of potential volunteers might find it necessary to take paying jobs. Any disturbance of the humanitarian-fiscal balance could have a critical impact.

Hospice care might succeed in its humanitarian agenda, then, and yet fail to secure a permanent place in the health- and social-services spectrum. Some experienced caregivers and administrators have also expressed concern that the terms of "success" might themselves lead to a degradation in hospice services. To improve its chances for fiscal survival, hospice care perhaps would lose its most distinguishing characteristics and increasingly come to resemble the more impersonal and mechanistic type of care that some believe is characteristic of the health-services establishment today.

Still another possibility has been envisioned. Assume that the hospice movement does succeed in both its humanitarian and its fiscal objectives. Might key elements of the hospice approach be applied to a broader spectrum of human services? Terminal illness is not the only condition in which effective use might be made of comfort and supportive care, an individual treatment program supervised by an interdisciplinary team, and utilization of skilled volunteers. Success of the hospice experiment in its initial sphere, then, might well encourage spin-off efforts in a variety of other need areas.

This chapter considers some of the major issues regarding public policy and the hospice movement, drawing upon results of the present study but also taking into account other findings and experiences. Particular attention will be given to the attempt to integrate the humane aims of the hospice approach with the economic and political milieu in which it functions.

How Should Hospice Research Influence Public Policy?

This issue deserves immediate attention because of its impact on all other issues affecting the hospice movement in the United States. Before federal entry into this area one might have identified the major possible relationships between policy formation and research and considered their respective merits. The alternatives, reduced to their essence, are:

1. to ignore research. Do what the people want—and do not offend any powerful constituencies.
2. to consult available research and not take any initiatives that are strongly contradicted by the data. The controlling principle, however, is still to act in accordance either with the grass-roots advocacy for support of the hospice approach, or in accordance with those opposed to such support: a political decision.
3. to provide additional support to research and evaluation efforts related to ongoing hospice organizations. Do not support hospice care or formulate

policy until all the findings are available and have been critically reviewed.

4. to do systematic research and evaluation, but not to delay policy formation until the findings are in hand. One option is to provide limited and temporary support for hospice programs and subsequently examine the process and outcomes. Another option is to restrict the limited and temporary support to existing medical centers for expanded home terminal-care programs rather than underwrite an experiment with the full-spectrum hospice approach.

Each of these alternatives implies a distinctively different orientation toward the role of evaluation research in policy formation. The history of twentieth-century political administration suggests that styles of decision making have continued to change. In the early 1950s, for example, a determined attempt was made to cast public administration into the mold of political science in response to "icy intellectual critiques" of public decision makers (Henry 1986, 29). From a practical standpoint, however, the effort to convert policy formation to a branch of science was not a striking success. The gap between the academic laboratory and "real life" was all too evident. As a form of compromise, the case-study method became increasingly popular. Policy decisions were to be made with rigorous scientific standards as background, but for practical purposes it might be sufficient to develop case-study reports that illuminated "questions of moral choice and decision-making behavior in the administrative milieu" (30). Even while the political science trend in policy formation and public administration was having its turn, a powerful counterforce appeared. The managerial approach gained in strength as the political science approach foundered. The world of commerce became the dominant frame of reference, with experts in business becoming dominant over political scientists. Decisions were to be made by the application of business principles—managerial expertise being more important than familiarity with particular substantive areas.

The scientific-versus-managerial dialectic was still much in evidence when in 1970 the federal government introduced a new emphasis on evaluating health-care programs with the passage of Section 513 of the Public Health Service Act. This measure authorized the spending of up to 1 percent of the Act's appropriation for evaluation grants and contracts. Section 513 also opened a new set of questions for the federal government regarding evaluation priorities and methods. As Abert (1979, 99) observed, there have been frequent discrepancies between congressional appropriations targeted for program evaluation "and the amount actually spent for this program." Lively controversy has arisen regarding the effectiveness of federal evaluation efforts, including what some have seen as the failure to identify the questions whose answers would have the most impact upon program decisions.

The decision to evaluate hospice programs and evaluate them in a particular way cannot be separated, then, either from the policy-making styles dominant at the moment or from the history and current status of the federal government's general health-evaluation program. What actually did happen?

The NHS and Its Use

Hospice care forced itself upon the national policy agenda on the basis of vigorous advocacy by patients, families, and health-care professionals, further amplified and articulated by the National Hospice Organization. The unifying motive was to improve the life of dying people and their families. Although this unquestionably was the dominant motive, a variety of other needs and desires expressed themselves through the hospice movement. Some health-care professionals who felt themselves to be suffering under the yoke of an overbearing and unresponsive medical profession saw in the hospice movement the opportunity to establish a more egalitarian relationship. The physician would be an important member of the interdisciplinary team, but no longer (or so it was hoped) an autocrat who exercised authority even in those areas where others had greater competence. A very different motive could also be detected: the entrepreneurial opportunity of developing chains of profit-making hospices. Still another motive (at least as suspected by some members of the health-care establishment) was that the federal government was interested in using hospice care as a kind of hammer to shatter the existing power structure. Hospital systems as well as physicians might be forced to function in new ways and become more amenable to cost containment and regulatory pressures in general. The reality behind motives as different as these cannot be determined with any real accuracy. The point, however, is that such motives were *perceived* by various parties to the hospice movement and its evaluation and contributed to the ever-shifting mélange from the first plans to data utilization.

Program evaluation was not likely to survive as a purely scientific (or "icily intellectual") venture within the force field sketched above. In fact, *Congress passed and signed legislation before the National Hospice Study was completed—despite the fact that this study had been requested by Congress specifically to assess the need for legislation.* This was certainly an odd sequence if one assumes a completely rational managerial or political science model of policy formation. It would not have been surprising, however, to those familiar with political realities. Research was not ignored, however. NHS findings did find application in the development of regulations, and the study was influential in shaping the system that emerged. Referring back to the alternatives listed above, the actual course of events most closely resembled the fourth option: "Do systematic research and evaluation, but do not delay policy formation until the findings are in hand." Furthermore, Congress took the more liberal of the two pathways within this option—supporting an evaluation of full-spectrum hospice services rather than a scaled-down version limited to existing medical center models.

Suppose, however, that Congress had instead decided to wait until completion of the NHS and had then based its decisions exclusively upon these findings. What would have happened? It is possible that Medicare support might not have been made available for a new system of care under the rubric of "hospice." The results did not demonstrate the sweeping superiority that many believe to be characteristic of the hospice approach, although hospice care does emerge generally in a positive light. Policy makers could have shied away from the complexities of the findings. The decision could have been made not to support a new system of care in return for which major improvements in outcome would be difficult to document. (Pain control, for an important example, continues to be a difficult although very relevant area in which to compare different approaches, because of problems inherent in the assessment of subjective states of being.) Rather than support hospices as an independent program, Congress could have elected to encourage hospicelike approaches within the conventional-care system, for example, increase funding of home-care and family-support services. This is not what happened. The political forces appeared to be decisive, and decisively in favor of hospices. Passage in 1982 of the Tax Equity and Fiscal Responsibility Act (TEFRA) did not require an extensive debate regarding cost reduction or other outcomes. Although this decision did not run counter to available data on hospice costs, it did run ahead of the major study commissioned by Congress itself.

The Medicare-supported system created by Congress contained something for most of the hospice proponents, if not always to the extent desired by various constituencies. For entrepreneurs, it established new opportunities in the increasingly competitive health-care system. Indeed, the legislation permits reimbursement of for-profit hospices that did not exist at the time and have only recently started to appear. For professional caregivers other than physicians, the law mandates interdisciplinary team control of patient care. Reimbursements are made only for care specifically ordered by the team. The hegemony of the M.D.s is thus threatened, although the final story has yet to be told. For taxpayers, the prospective payment system and fiscal cap on total stay ($6,500 in final regulations) are included as evidence of fiscal control and responsibility. The per diem rates, however, have already been adjusted upward twice under pressure from providers and can be expected to be subjected to annual negotiations. Volunteers, pastoral counselors, and other providers are assured of their roles by having their participation required as a condition for Medicare certification. The result, then, was a politically oriented distributive legislative act that created a reimbursement program that may differ substantially from the movement that spawned it.

Almost lost in a new mix of federal requirements and opportunities are the smaller, volunteer-oriented organizations that have contributed greatly to the establishment and early success of hospice care in the United States. The increasingly commercialized and competitive environment made possible by

Congress could prove a severe challenge to the survival of the very hospices whose pioneering efforts provided the core of the movement.

Continued study and surveillance of Medicare-reimbursed hospice care has been ordered by Congress. Hospice support could have been withdrawn in keeping with the "sunset" provision embedded in the original legislation. However, Congress ensured that Medicare would not withdraw support for hospice care, regardless of the results of continued study, by eliminating that provision of the law in 1985. Financial support for human service systems, once established, is extremely difficult to terminate. Furthermore, hospice care remains an attractive alternative in terminal care for a significant segment of the American public, and in our pluralistic society, alternatives are easily justifiable when they have strong support from special-interest groups. It is perhaps one of the hospice movement's most notable distinctions that its "special" interests pertain to one of the most universal of interests—to live in comfort and dignity in the face of death.

In retrospect, it can be seen that those responsible for hospice policy formation recognized the need for systematic program evaluation but were not prepared to accept a cut-and-dried relationship between data and decision making. Political judgment as well as technical information was required in developing public policy regarding an area that was both as personal and sensitive as terminal care and as frought with economic and power issues as the health-care industry. Theoretically, the study could have been strengthened by independence from such political factors as predetermined choice of participating hospice organizations. But the decision makers could also have been even less mindful of the need for objective data. The shaping and support of the NHS by Congress might well be considered an example of politics as the art of compromise.

Some Policy Implications for the Health-Care System

The emergence of hospice care as a viable alternative for terminally ill individuals and their families raises a number of health policy and organizational issues regarding the delivery of health care. These issues relate to the function and operation of hospices, the role of the physician, the social responsibility of family members, and a host of other major social and health policies. What follows is a discussion of some of these policy issues, drawing upon NHS findings.

Who Chooses Hospice Care?

Cancer was the primary diagnosis of more than 90 percent of the thirteen thousand patients who were admitted to the forty hospices participating in the NHS. People with terminal conditions other than cancer had longer stays and higher and more variable costs, on the average. Most hospice patients (again, over 90 percent) had strong social supports, usually family, living with and assisting the patient in the tasks of daily living. Despite the availability of Medicare reimbursement in demonstration hospices, relatively few patients (under 10 percent) lived alone, and substantially higher costs were incurred for the care of these people. The overall results of the NHS might have been quite different had more noncancer patients and those without family support entered hospice care. Patients lacking family support might benefit greatly from the hospice approach, but one cannot assume that the cost consequences would be comparable. With the increasing visibility of the hospice approach, it is possible that more people with conditions other than cancer and more people with limited family support will be interested in this option. It may be that national policy modifications will be necessary to assist local hospice organizations in making decisions that are both humane and fiscally viable.

When the hospice choice is made seems to be almost as important as the characteristics of the person who makes it. NHS data show that a high proportion of patients make the choice for hospice care very late in the course of their illness. Frequently the choice is made just prior to death. Although the average length of stay in the NHS (*participation* might be the more appropriate term) varied across hospices from just over fifty days to over a hundred days, the median length of stay was fairly uniform at around thirty-five days. Patients, families, and providers appear to be electing hospice admission at a fairly late point. This pattern could be seen as constituting a very appropriate utilization of the hospice resource. After having exhausted all possible curative means, patients may seek relief in the palliation offered by hospice care. An alternative interpretation is also possible, however. Some physicians may be reluctant to recommend hospice care until near the end. In the absence of adequate research on this topic (see chapter 13), one is left with the possibility that hospice care does not have the opportunity to do all it can for some patients and families because of a bias toward late referrals.

NHS quality-of-life analyses suggest that delay in selecting the hospice alternative may reduce or eliminate the benefits hospice care was designed to provide. It is important to note, however, that the hospice movement has been vulnerable to criticism that patients may select this option too soon and therefore fail to receive remission-oriented treatment. NHS data indicate a marked tendency toward late, as opposed to early, admissions, and hospice leaders such as London's Dr. Cicely Saunders have often attempted to provide reassurance regarding their hospices' alertness to opportunities for more aggressive treatment when indicated. The "when" issue sits atop competing views of hospice aims and operation. It would be useful if the conflicting opinions on timing of hospice admission could be resolved not only by follow-up research but by the willingness of all parties to examine their views in the light of the available data.

How to decide when the patient should be referred, and who should participate in that decision, is a major issue related to the role of hospices in the larger health-care system. This challenge may be even more pertinent when the terminal condition (or configuration of conditions) is other than cancer. The possibility of premature hospice admission raises ethical as well as organizational and financial issues in the presence of chronic diseases whose terminal course has not been defined adequately. As long as a clear and reliable concept of "the terminal phase" is lacking for a particular life-threatening condition, all those involved in decision making will continue to cope with uncertainty in deciding "when." Advocates of aggressive medical care at times even take the extreme position that "terminal illness" is a label that should never be used because it constitutes giving up hope. Advocates of the palliative approach have been known to counter this stance with the charge that an aggressive medical approach that does not know its own limits is fueled by a strong component of anxiety and denial and deprives patient and family of the opportunity for a dignified and personally meaningful final phase of life. Policy makers are not likely to resolve this conflict, but they certainly should be aware of both sides in the continuing dialectic.

Physicians in Hospices and Traditional-Care Settings

Physician utilization in the NHS was greater for nonhospice patients. The lowest level of physician utilization occurred among home-care hospice patients (who also spent the fewest days in an inpatient setting). Approximately 80 percent of reported physicians' visits to demonstration hospice patients were made by their primary physician. This finding suggests that the physicians did *not* abandon their patients after making the referral to a hospice. The possibility of abandonment has been raised in the minds of some observers by the tendency of physicians to neglect patients after admission to nursing homes. Although the NHS data are encouraging in this respect, there remains the danger that under some circumstances physicians will abdicate their responsibilities once the patient is referred to a hospice. If hospice referral is perceived as an act equivalent to pulling the plug, then patients actively referred by physicians may be predominately those who will have very short stays (seven days or less); this subgroup comprised almost 20 percent of admissions to NHS hospices. Physicians who are averse to working within the interdisciplinary team framework as well as those unwilling or unable to face dying patients might be expected to behave in this manner. Similarly, the physician who reluctantly approves the hospice alternative because of family and patient pressure may also be tempted to withdraw from the picture.

The physician's role in communicating to patients and families about disease prognosis may also influence both the decision and its timing. A substantial literature has developed regarding the ways in which physicians inform patients of their prognosis and how the patients' understanding of their disease influences treatment choices. In the NHS, a minimum of 15 percent of hospice patients denied the presence of metastatic disease around the time of entry—in spite of the fact that demonstration hospices required patient-signed consent stipulating that the prognosis was six months or less. It is not known how much of this attitude of denial, if any, resulted from problems in physician-patient communication. The correlates and consequences of denial are far from simple (e.g., Breznitz 1983). Nevertheless, physicians and other caregivers might be well advised to be attentive to patients' (and families') perceptions. Policy makers perhaps should recognize that it may be adaptive for some people to interpret their conditions at variance with the medical realities, and therefore should not impose confrontational regulations. The hospice philosophy does not insist that patients acknowledge and accept their prognosis at admission.

The hospice approach is to provide health and social services to patients and their families through the organizational means of an interdisciplinary team. Physicians as a group are not comfortable working within democratic structures such as interdisciplinary care-planning teams. This may explain why physician utilization was lower in the hospice settings as compared with the traditional-care settings. Why this difference exists, however, cannot be determined from the available information. It is reasonable to hypothesize, however, that the traditional primary physician would find it more difficult to operate within an environment in which he or she was not the unquestioned authority. Perhaps primary-care physicians are not willing to devote the amount of time required by the interdisciplinary team approach. The available information is not sufficient to confirm these suspicions, but the physician may withdraw from involvement both in terms of physical presence and psychological attitude. The enduring success of hospice care may depend to some extent on gradual attitudinal changes among experienced physicians and on an increase in the number of new physicians who see family and allied health professionals as integral partners.

The legal liability of primary physicians, given the hospice team's role in determining care, is another important issue that must be considered. According to most state laws, it is the physician who prescribes, and it is on the authority of the physician's signature that other services are arranged—regardless of the participatory process undertaken in reaching the decision. The practice implications of the first hospice malpractice suits may be considerable, and such suits are likely in our litigious society.

The Family Role as Hospice Care Providers

If hospice care is cost-effective, it is because the family bears much of the cost. Home care appears to be feasible only when the family "pays" for the patient's presence at home by providing many hours of direct care. This cost shifting from the formal to the informal system is consistent with other recent health policies such as early hospital discharge and "same-day surgery." These alterations in the locus of care require both the willingness and the ability of families to assume the care burden at home. Some potential family caregivers have strong commitments but are unable to carry them out because of other significant competing responsibilities or their own physical frailty. It is unfair to assume that those who do not provide home care have a lack of affection or willingness to help. In the case of elderly cancer patients, for example, the next of kin often is an elderly person with several major physical problems that reduce the energy available for helping one's disabled spouse on a day-by-day basis.

The willingness of hospice families to assume their strenuous role is not necessarily applicable to the typical long-term-care patient population. Families of cancer patients with relatively time-limited prognoses will temporarily coalesce around the caretaking responsibilities that have been thrust upon them. This level of commitment is difficult to sustain over a period of many years, as is often the case in the long-term care of people with illnesses other than cancer. Increasing the number of noncancer hospice patients whose lengths of stay may be substantially longer than the median hospice patient's could result in an intolerable strain on other family members. And once families exceed their ability to provide the needed support at home, the more costly inpatient setting often becomes the only alternative.

The people caring for patients in home-based hospice programs had to provide exceptionally high levels of support for their stricken family members—much more than was required of those whose kin were served by hospital-based hospices. Nevertheless, the perceptions of burden reported by primary care persons in the home-care situation was only slightly higher. Furthermore, there were no consistent differences between caregivers in both settings with respect to secondary morbidity. Those providing care in home-based programs did not themselves suffer a higher rate of hospitalization or make excessive use of alcohol, medication, or physician visits. This suggests that the increased burden assumed by families did not necessarily result in social or physical dysfunction, at least in the short term.

Hospital Role and Hospice Care

In the National Hospice Study, nineteen of the forty participating hospices were classified as hospital-based. This proportion is consistent with data from a 1982 Joint Commission of Hospital Accreditation survey of hospice programs around the United States. Nearly half of all programs responding were affiliated with institutions having an inpatient unit. The vast majority of these hospital-based hospices (to our knowledge) are incorporated within not-for-profit institutions. Why hospitals have chosen to become involved in providing hospice care is of considerable interest. Most of the eleven hospital-based demonstration hospices experienced difficulties in allocating costs unequivocally to a hospice "cost center." This accounting requirement was not imposed on non-demonstration hospices, some of which reserved beds for hospice use and tolerated occasional low utilization rates. In all instances, hospitals were willing to devote extra staff time resources to their hospice units. Our analyses of hospice inpatient unit costs revealed that this additional staff time led to higher routine per diem costs than was the case for nonhospice inpatient beds. On the other hand, in most inpatient hospices, the level of ancillary services used per inpatient day by hospice patients was markedly lower than that for comparable terminal conventional-care patients.

Why are such higher-cost hospice units established and maintained by hospitals? This question assumes increased importance in view of the prospective payment reimbursement system introduced by Medicare. Hospitals might be expected to lack interest in creating hospices within their facilities because the costs per bed could be expected to exceed those for a comparable nonhospice bed. The low utilization of ancillary services—a major source of revenue for most hospitals—would also be expected to reduce the hospital revenues per inpatient day when hospice patients are added to the overall patient census.

Given these disincentives, why should a hospital establish a hospice unit? Certain hypotheses can be advanced, although an extensive econometric marketing-and-demand analysis is required to address this question adequately. First, some professional staff and members of boards of directors may have themselves become advocates of the hospice approach. The normal "bottom line" thinking that prevails in corporate decision making may have been set aside because key participants saw an opportunity to introduce a program of exceptional social value. Representing the community at large, hospital board members could see hospice involvement as an appropriate expression of the hospital's larger mission.

Alternatively (but not necessarily in contradiction to the humanitarian position), it could be hypothesized that some hospitals may have chosen to offer hospice services as a "loss leader." The first hospital in a particular locale to establish a successful hospice program might, by so doing, gain perceived superiority in corporate image. Similar to "one-stop shopping," a medical center could promote itself as serving a broad range of needs from intensive medical care to inpatient palliation. Hospice inpatient units might be seen as more desirable and therefore become more prevalent in areas where there are surplus beds in acute hospitals. Empty beds are converted to hospice beds in a "goodwill" maneuver. This is more than a gesture, because new and valuable services are provided—and empty beds generate even less revenue than hospice beds.

Perhaps the most important issues regarding the involvement of acute care hospitals in hospice care are related to the definition of acute palliative care. Hospice inpatient care entails a higher staff-patient ratio but a reduced use of costly ancillary tests and procedures. If the difference between hospice care and conventional care is merely one of the increased nursing time, then the locus of care might well be shifted from the hospital to less technologically intensive chronic disease and/or skilled nursing facilities. If the low use of invasive procedures and diagnostic tests observed in the NHS is the norm for hospice care, then one can question the appropriateness of the acute care hospital as the locus of palliative care.

Fifty years ago, more than 80 percent of American deaths occurred at home. Since the early 1950s, there has been an increasing "medicalization" of terminal illness to the point that by 1979, only 13.7 percent of all cancer deaths occurred in a home, and only an additional 20 percent occurred in a nonacute institutional setting. Having molded social values to favor the acute hospital for the provision of terminal care, it is unlikely that the hospital industry will relinquish control of a patient population that accounts for a disproportionate percentage of all hospital bed days. If the acute hospital disguised as a hospice becomes the locus of care for terminal patients—"winning out" against the home or some other alternative palliative-care setting—then a personal and social phenomenon will have been rather decisively transformed into a "medical" one. This battle for the terminal patient is still in progress, however, and is being fought primarily in the long-term arena. Control over health and medical-care practice is being disputed among physicians, hospitals, and the nursing and home-care world. The outcome of this struggle will greatly influence not only the process of care itself, but also the future definition of terminal care.

The Twilight of American Voluntarism?

The emergence of hospices as a component of the health-care establishment raises the specter of professionalizing one of the last bastions of traditional voluntary activity in the United States. The introduction of new professional roles such as volunteer coordinators and bereavement counselors forces us to ask whether hospices will supplement or supplant the traditional functions undertaken by volunteer associations in communities across the nation. Unfortunately, history does not favor voluntarism when reimbursement arrangements are introduced. For example, with the advent of Medicare and Medicaid, many hospitals and physicians eliminated the free care they had provided to the indigent population before insurance became available. Will voluntary clergy and/or volunteer groups be crowded out of the hospice movement to be replaced by professional bereavement counselors and grief-abatement programs? And would such an outcome be particularly devastating because volunteers have been so important to the hospice movement, thereby contributing to a more general demise of voluntarism?

From the larger perspective, the emergence of hospice care can be envisioned as yet another step in the "institutionalization" of certain social functions traditionally carried out by the family. Providing care and emotional support to family members following the death of a loved one has long been viewed as a family responsibility. With the medical formalization of the hospice movement, society's perception of what is appropriate familial responsibility and behavior may change, perhaps leading to a uniform institutionalized approach to death and dying. This would represent an unfortunate further "homogenization" of American life.

Qualitative and anecdotal data obtained during the NHS suggest that the hospice leadership structure is already shifting from broad community consumer representation to a standard type of executive board in which professionals dominate. Volunteerism remains alive and well, but a trend toward professionalization can also be noted and may prove to have important policy implications in the years ahead.

Legislative Implications of the National Hospice Study

The Tax Equity and Fiscal Responsibility Act (TEFRA) was passed in the summer of 1982, at a time when knowledge of hospice programs and their pattern of care was still rudimentary. The pioneering legislation reflected the input of a coalition of hospice advocates, most of whom advocated a home-care orientation that was consistent with the cost-saving argument. Following passage of this legislation, the policy-development staff of the Health Care Financing Administration (HCFA) prepared regulations intended to facilitate the application of the new law. As already noted, these regulations were influenced by preliminary data from the NHS.

This section raises a series of questions emanating from our review of the TEFRA legislation and the associated regulations within the context of NHS findings.

The hospice provisions of the TEFRA legislation and the regulations promulgated from them comprise a complex interlocking set of incentives and constraints that HCFA believes remain true to the legislative intent. Briefly, the law and regulations define "terminally ill" eligible patients as those certified as having a life expectancy of six months or less. A total of three benefit periods, the first two of ninety days each and the third of thirty days, constitute an individual's lifetime eligibility for the hospice benefit. Once the patient has become a hospice beneficiary, he or she waives all rights to Medicare reimbursement under the regular Medicare system while receiving hospice benefits.

To be eligible for participation in the program, hospices must also meet certain conditions. The availability of a core staff is among these conditions. The core must include qualified personnel representing nursing, medicine, medical social services, and counseling. Through its medical director the hospice must assume comprehensive responsibility for all aspects of the patient-care program. Another condition of participation is that hospices must give assurance that no more than 20 percent of the total patient days of hospice care in a year will be provided in an inpatient setting. The entire set of regulations is lengthy and detailed, representing a substantial degree of control over any hospice organization that would participate in the reimbursement program.

The reimbursement formula itself is innovative. A different prospective rate is specified for each of four types of "days of care." The principal types of hospice day are classified as "routine home care" and "general inpatient care." Two additional types of care are available in principle—inpatient respite (offering temporary relief to the caregiving family), and continuous home-care days that are reimbursed in blocks of eight hours. There is an overall Medicare-imposed cap of $6,500 on the average per-patient cost that a hospice organization can incur in the course of any given year. Hospices are also responsible for paying 100 percent of the reasonable services for physician services furnished by hospice employees or by physicians working under arrangement with the hospice. Primary-care physicians are paid 80 percent of reasonable charges under the regular Part B Medicare program. Individual patients are not liable for any hospice-care services, with the exception of a 5 percent coinsurance payment for drugs and biologicals provided on an outpatient basis and inpatient respite care. However, the patient is responsible for any medical services that might be provided without express permission of the hospice interdisciplinary clinical team.

The checks and balances inherent in the legislation and regulations are not appreciated in their full complexity unless one has some experience with the existing pattern of hospice utilization. Participating hospices are continually challenged to meet patient needs and at the same time survive financially. Clinical expertise is necessary but not sufficient. The hospice that falters in its balancing act between mix of patients enrolled and mix of services provided is in some danger of becoming an ex-hospice. Despite its merits, the present reimbursement system creates a constant hazard for hospice survival, no matter how effective the hospice may be in meeting its primary-care objectives. Hospices must admit patients whose needs can be met within the $6,500 average patient cap and who will spend less than 20 percent of their patient days in an inpatient setting. At the same time, patients are needed who will spend days at home without requiring any home services. Such patient days build a revenue base to compensate for those individuals who require more resources per day than the revenue their days generate. All this requires very careful patient selection and equally careful management of services and financial resources. Hospice care has entered the health-care establishment at a price: intensive fiscal control and frequently burdensome regulations that may have serious implications for its progress and its viability.

Core Services

Hospices participating in the NHS did not necessarily provide all the core services directly. Some hospices served primarily as coordinating agencies, contracting with existing home health agencies for services. This approach has largely been eliminated by the requirement that federal reimbursement will be made only to hospices that provide essentially all the core services themselves. (This provision has been modified to exempt rural hospices.) The requirement for direct services may have had the advantage of encouraging the development of stronger and more comprehensive hospice organizations—but it may also result in the duplication of services and an additional cost to the overall health-care system in various areas.

Patient Selection

Patient selection is perhaps the most important decision that hospices must face in their daily operations. Too many patients staying "too long" (in the fiscal, not necessarily the clinical, sense) may result in the hospice's exceeding the $6,500 average per-patient cap. On the other hand, patients who on admission are extremely ill and require intensive resources will have short lengths of stay without generating commensurate levels of revenue. Very difficult situations can arise: if a hospice accepts home-care patients with acute resource-intensive problems, then the unreimbursed expense could jeopardize the organization's continued viability. And yet how can such patients be ethically rejected when it is clear the family caregivers cannot cope with these needs in the home? Those responsible for reviewing hospice policy should give serious attention to this kind of repeated dilemma.

Hospices might select only the least costly patients with the most predictable courses. If most hospices decided to behave in this manner, then the population of potentially eligible patients for the hospice benefit would be considerably smaller than initial estimates have suggested. This approach might well expose hospices to humanitarian criticism. Furthermore, by reducing the number of acceptable patients, the smaller constituency could fail to support the number of hospices that have emerged across America.

Service Mix

A condition of participation for hospices, as already noted, is that no more than 20 percent of the aggregate number of hospice patient days during any year be spent in an inpatient setting. Furthermore, exceeding this limit of inpatient days is likely to raise average per-patient costs above the $6,500 cap unless this is offset by the number of very-short-stay patients. This creates a potentially dangerous scenario. Theoretically, hospices could serve as "dumping grounds" for hospitals and nursing homes, accepting many very-short-stay patients for the fiscal advantages involved. It is important to recognize that the 20 percent cap on the proportion of inpatient days is not a reimbursement constraint but rather a provision that is required as a basic condition of participation.

How reasonable is this condition in light of available data? NHS findings indicate that for participating home-care hospices, only 8 percent of "hospice days" were spent in an inpatient setting. This figure is well below the 20 percent upper limit. The pattern is quite different, however, for hospital-based hospices. Patients admitted to hospital-based hospices spent 28 percent of their time in inpatient settings. Furthermore, more than a third of hospital-based patients were *always* in an inpatient setting. It is likely that inpatient hospices tend to have a distinctive type of patient mix. Somewhere between a third and a half of all hospital-based hospice patients might never spend a day at home. Another 20 percent might have very long stays at hospices, but mostly at home, while the remaining 30 percent would have an average length of stay with an average number of inpatient days as well. This mix could support the survival of hospital-based hospices. A large number of days at home for a small number of patients might more than compensate for the large proportion of patients who spend all of their short time in hospice within an inpatient setting.

Similarly, there are dynamics associated with maintaining patients at home by buttressing the existing informal support system. The home-care day reimbursement rates developed by HCFA were based on utilization patterns for the delivery of home care provided by hospital-based and home care–based hospices. In the NHS, short-stay patients had higher per–home day costs than did long-stay patients. Long-stay patients were more likely to have days in which no services were delivered. Shorter-stay patients in a home-care setting were provided more intensive care because they were usually close to death. Hospices in the future will have to assess very carefully the revenue generated by home days and the level of services provided to patients while at home. Patients with stronger available family support usually require fewer services. Consequently, the cost of patients with strong families will be relatively low, while the revenue they generate will be equivalent to the revenue generated by high-cost patients. Hospice organizations concerned about their fiscal survival might understandably utilize a "strength of family support" indicator as a criterion for entry.

In order to balance the cost and revenue dynamics, hospices may have to limit the cost of the service mix they provide by increasing the number of lower-cost staff. Home health aides and homemakers might be more likely to provide care on standard home-care days, whereas nursing services would become increasingly important as the patient's physiological problems are exacerbated in the final weeks of life. This approach to cost containment might also be subject to criticism, however, by those who hold that professional competency would be compromised.

Clinical and Fiscal Control

Controlling the pattern of care is the responsibility of the interdisciplinary clinical team. This responsibility includes both the clinical and the fiscal. Outpatient clinic visits, diagnostic tests, consultations by specialists, and—most saliently—inpatient procedures all represent costs borne by the hospice. The exercise of control is a key to projecting hospice behavior in the future. Maintaining fiscal and clinical control while patients are in an inpatient setting is a major concern. In the NHS, hospices with their own inpatient units had substantially lower ancillary costs per patient day than was the case for those admitted to standard acute-care hospitals. Under the demonstration, HC hospices were not required to control ancillary service use or inpatient costs. However, hospice directors reported feeling responsible for controlling the clinical care provided in the hospital setting. Under TEFRA, control may have to be increased to ensure that home-care hospices will have a viable and fiscally stable arrangement with an inpatient setting.

Inpatient care need not take place in an acute hospital. It is conceivable that other settings could meet the inpatient hospice requirement. NHS patients made very limited use of skilled nursing facilities. This form of service was rarely used despite the fact that demonstration sites did have the option to contract for inpatient respite care. In the future more consideration will probably be given to developing effective relationships between the hospice and the labor-intensive palliative-care unit within a skilled nursing facility. Among the potential hazards, however, is the removal of the terminally ill patient (and hospice) from the mainstream of the medical-care system.

A final question emerging from our analysis of TEFRA in light of NHS data is whether the legislation and its regulations meet the originally identified social need as articulated by the hospice movement. Establishing a separate system of care could lead to hospices' becoming classified as another form of the not highly esteemed nursing home industry. This would be unfortunate, since one of the original goals of the hospice movement was to act as a catalyst upon the existing system. The legislation may also lead to professionalization of the current voluntary aspects of the hospice movement. Part of the hospice mystique, at least in the United States, was to have families, communities, and lay people actively involved in the recognition and acceptance of terminal illness. This voluntary community base may still have much to contribute, and its possible replacement by a professional approach deserves careful reevaluation.

Some Concluding Thoughts

Some key issues confronting the hospice movement have been examined. Public advocacy for this alternative approach to terminal care found a responsive chord in Congress. Legislation authorizing a Medicare-associated reimbursement system was enacted while the National Hospice Study was still in progress, but the findings were consulted in the subsequent development of regulations. The rapid growth of hospice care in the United States and its equally rapid entry into the federal reimbursement-and-regulatory apparatus suggest that hospice care is perceived as meeting a significant sociomedical need.

Nevertheless, all those involved with hospices face the challenge of performing a difficult balancing act, with the long-term outcome far from certain. The federal government's role includes balancing the elements of (1) support, (2) quality assurance, and (3) fiscal responsibility. Each of these components has, in fact, been given systematic attention: the reimbursement plan is operational, exacting criteria have been established to ensure that participating hospices meet standards, and mechanisms such as a benefit cap and a limitation on the number of inpatient hospice days have been put into place to control expenditures. It would have been remarkable if this system had emerged as a perfect set of checks and balances. The hospice experiment has some novel structural aspects along with its innovative philosophy and service delivery. To accommodate the still-evolving hospice movement, it may be advisable to ensure a realistic match between clinical needs, hospice operation, and fiscal guidelines. It would be unfortunate if the reimbursement system should damage the movement itself.

NHS data as well as other studies and experiences indicate that the hospice movement in general has performed well in comparison with the alternatives. At the very least, those who have selected hospices do not seem to have suffered any deprivation of care, have often (although not in all instances) required a lower level of expenditure, and have usually been able to spend more time at home. Furthermore, the hospice movement, with its emphasis on the interdisciplinary team, individualization of care, and utilization of volunteers, stands as a potential model for other health-care applications. Hospice experience has potential for introducing physicians to a productive interdisciplinary team approach that could flourish in other settings as well.

Perhaps the essential question that policy makers must ask themselves (and the data) is the following: "With the advent of hospice care, has the health-care system become more responsive to the needs and desires of Americans?" Advocates and critics alike deserve a clear-cut answer.

13

Concepts, Questions, and Research Priorities

DAVID S. GREER,
VINCENT MOR,
AND ROBERT KASTENBAUM

Hospice Care as a Manifestation of Sociocultural Change

Hospice care is both a service program and a social phenomenon. It is the product of an era and will flourish only if it continues to be consistent with social and professional trends. In this final chapter we briefly review the factors that influenced the emergence of hospices and discuss the implications of these forces for the future of hospice care in the United States.

Hospices arose at a time of increasing health-care cost consciousness. The ebullient expansiveness of Western societies post–World War II was replaced during the 1970s by a growing awareness of economic limitations, and nowhere more so than in the health-care arena. The health-care segment of the consumer price index rose nearly 20 percent per year in the mid 1970s as the Medicaid and Medicare entitlement programs expanded access to their beneficiaries, primarily the aged and poor. In addition, as exemplified by the End-Stage Renal Disease Program, whose cost exceeded estimates by nearly twenty times, providing access to new technology often produced runaway entitlement costs.

Simultaneously, the limitations and negative implications of scientific and technologic development were increasingly recognized. The promised miracle cures of cancer and heart disease remained remote despite expensive scientific "wars" on these diseases and others. The utopian leisure society, raised to expect the miracles of modern science to transform life and death, became increasingly frustrated with technology amid concern about nuclear annihilation, environmental pollution, and other adverse societal phenomena attributed to scientific "advance."

The stage was set for a return to traditional values and humanistic philosophies; self-care, the family, community, voluntarism, and personal autonomy were recalled as elements of the "good old days." Hospices reminded people that care was as important as cure, especially when the latter remained elusive despite aggressive, invasive, painful, and often humiliating scientifically based interventions. Hospices recalled that care of the sick and dying was a valued and respected vocation prior to the advent of science and that it was provided by families, neighbors, and practitioners with little, if any, scientific expertise.

It was no accident that the hospice movement arose in Western societies that were committed to individual autonomy, as opposed to the autocracy of the Eastern, socialized nations; hospice care was an expression of commitment to personal freedom rather than submission to authority, whether political or professional. The focus on personal autonomy was consistent with the orientation of those moving away from technology. Consumer choice became a rallying call for advocates of alternate approaches to the conventional practice of medicine.

Hospice care was also consistent with demographic trends. Population aging brought with it a shift in disease prevalence from acute to chronic. Death became predominantly a phenomenon associated with aging rather than infancy and childhood, as it had been historically. Chronic diseases rather than infectious diseases became the most common causes. In the United States as well as in many other industrialized societies, the growing population sixty-five years of age and older amplified the trend toward chronic-disease prevalence. An increasingly large percentage of the population had one or more chronic diseases. Many types of cancer have their peak incidence after the age of sixty-five. The incidence and mortality rates of colon, breast, and prostate cancer all peak among older persons; over 10 percent of persons over seventy have had a diagnosis of cancer (Feldman et al. 1986).

The increasing population of the aged and infirm requires greater commitment to health care from society, particularly from the family. Geographic and social mobility of the U.S. population since the end of World War II has diminished the capacity of the family to meet the needs of an increasingly dependent population. These gaps in the social-support network were likely to be filled in a manner that was consistent with humanistic and anti-institutional social trends. The burgeoning home health industry of the last fifteen years has been ample testimony to the demand for assistance in maintaining the independence of those in need.

Hospice care was, of course, not the only response to these sociocultural forces. The U.S. health-care system in general shifted rapidly toward home and self-care and away from hospital and institutional care and continues to do so at an accelerating pace (see figure 13.1). Throughout most of the twentieth century the predominant trend in health care has been toward increasingly institutional and technological sophistication. In figure 13.1 this translates into a gradual shift away from the self, family, and indigenous practitioners such as the

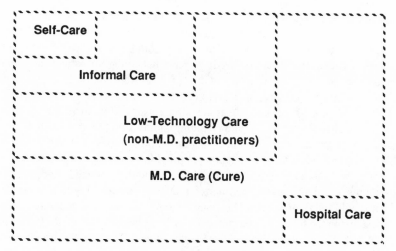

Figure 13.1   Health Care Alternatives

midwife to the curatively oriented physician practicing in the cathedral of medicine, the hospital. Over the past decade this trend has begun to reverse itself. These shifts in the pattern of care have been paralleled to a certain extent by shifts in where decedents die. The proportion of persons with cancer dying at home decreased during the first half of the century, reaching a nadir at around 13 percent in 1979. This trend was reversed in the first half of the current decade such that in some areas nearly 30 percent of cancer deaths are occurring at home. All of the trends noted above were active in promoting a "deinstitutional" approach to health-care delivery, with increasing emphasis on the role of family and home care. These trends have been accentuated recently by the impact of cost constraints.

In summary, vigorous and public opposition to "extraordinary" interventions for the prolongation of life, the growth of home and community-based care, including the massive deinstitutionalization programs in the mental-health field, strident calls for sharp reductions in health-care costs, particularly hospital costs, and the rise of "alternative" practitioners are all manifestations of the social forces that generated the hospice movement.

The Implications of These Changes

Hospices represent an opportunity to examine the broader and longer-term implications of current health-care trends. Like the scientific revolution that preceded it, the humanistic revolution will have both positive and negative aspects, and the balance will determine its long-term viability. Will hospices, and health care in general, continue to evolve in current directions? Or will disillusionment set in as the negatives become increasingly apparent? In the following we explore some of the issues that could impede the further development of hospices.

Hospice care has been able to meet the needs of the patients it cares for by shifting a large measure of the burden of care from the formal to the informal system, particularly the family. We have seen that caring for patients at home results in substantial loss of income of caregivers as well as considerable loss of leisure time that would otherwise have been devoted to other activities. Will the family of the future continue to bear the burden, particularly in view of the demographic changes, mobility, and changing family structure that are now occurring? Geographic mobility leaves increasing proportions of elderly with no children nearby who can be called upon to provide the in-home support so necessary in the U.S. hospices, which are highly home-care oriented. Recent census figures reveal that nearly one-quarter of all women over sixty-five are heads of households and can therefore be assumed to live alone. Current divorce rates suggest that in the future this proportion may be even higher. In the NHS, most terminal cancer patients in hospices lived with others. Demographic trends may shrink the pool of potential patients able to draw upon the social-support network that is vital for hospices to be able to meet their needs.

The response of the family to cancer patients has thus far been encouraging. Families have been more than willing to bear the burden of increased caretaking responsibility. We found that this increased burden had little effect on such "hard" measures of secondary morbidity as hospitalization, doctor use, alcoholism, and drug taking. There were indications that the primary caretakers of patients cared for by home-care hospices experienced more symptoms commonly associated with depression than was the case for helpers whose patients were cared for in an inpatient hospice. Our results also suggest that intensive commitment to home care over a protracted period does have an effect on the caretakers' ability to readjust after the patients' death.

The response of caregivers working in less predictable clinical situations such as Alzheimer's disease has not been as positive. Perhaps the prospects of a caretaking commitment of indefinite duration may make the burden all the more difficult to bear. A key issue that hospices will have to address in the future is whether families will continue to bear the burden needed to realize the benefits of hospice care, for cancer patients as well as those with diseases of less predictable durations. The tendency to increased home-care burden while the patient undergoes active treatment due to shifts toward ambulatory treatment, and strong incentives to reduce the length of hospital stay, may lead to family breakdown by the time the terminal phase approaches.

An element of missionary fervor seems necessary to maintain the voluntarism that characterizes and supports hospices. The original hospice advocates did battle with the sacred myths of curative medicine as well as the very powerful medical establishment. They set out to alter the pattern of medical care for the terminal cancer patient and ended up not only achieving that end but developing a parallel system that has flourished. These goals were achieved with the help of the intense commitment of community volunteers, teamed with disaffected medical and nursing professionals fully aware of the failings of the existing system. As the hospice movement has reached fruition and become institutionalized, the question of how this intense commitment of the hospice origins can be sustained must be addressed. Can the zeal of individuals as well as religious and secular sponsors be maintained? Since leadership in the hospice movement has so often emerged from the involved lay sector, will that same dynamism be present in a movement dominated by professionals, each with his or her own personal and professional agenda?

The hospice "team" introduced a new element of egalitarianism into health care. Team practice challenges the traditional dominion of the largely male medical profession. Similar trends are discernible in other health-care sectors, but nowhere are they more advanced or explicit than in hospices. We found that during an era of nursing shortages many of the most skilled and experienced specialists were seeking employment in hospices, which could pay them only a fraction of what established medical institutions could offer. The autonomy of action and equal footing with which nurses and other professionals function relative to physicians in the hospice environment was a significant attraction. To date, the relationship between physicians and nurses in hospices has been positive, largely because of the types of professionals drawn to this type of work. As the hospice of the future becomes more formalized, will power relationships impair team function? Can valid diagnostic and therapeutic decisions emerge from a group process? Or, as one cynical physician put it, can clinical decision making be based on a "one man, one vote" principle? The legal as well as the ethical implications of group decision making have yet to be tested. Language in the current Medicare hospice legislation suggests that the hospice interdisciplinary team, as a unit, is the final determinant of the patient's clinical care. Who participates in the "team," who is responsible for the decisions of the team, and who is sued if malpractice is claimed?

As we have indicated, hospice care reflects changing societal expectations of the health-care system, from cure to care, extension of life to quality of life. Quality of life is an ephemeral term, dependent on a myriad of personal value judgments, cultural orientations, and social considerations. How can one quantify or objectify such an elusive concept? Profound societal ethical values are raised by this type of valuing. Hospices will undoubtedly be at the center of these issues and controversies. Precisely because of the countless difficult ethical and professional decisions hospice staff will have to make, hospices may be an important barometer of shifting social mores and values; the survival of hospices may depend on their consistency with these trends.

The Role of Research in Policy Formulation

There is a large cultural gap between community leaders (politicians, bureaucrats, and others) and scientists; their values and needs differ markedly. What is the role of objective research in policy formulation? Whose needs are to be addressed? The politicians'? The scientists'? And what about the clinicians, who are responsible for delivering the care?

It must be conceded that health-service research is still in its infancy. There are numerous difficulties researchers face in conducting policy research on the costs and benefits of health-care programs, ranging from the methodologies and end points used to define program benefits to the complexities of communicating the results to the various interested constituencies.

In the National Hospice Study (NHS), the fundamental question of whether hospice care is a desirable approach to meeting the needs of the terminally ill appeared relatively simple, but answering it required the complexity that we have reviewed throughout this book. Policy makers seek definitive, immutable answers. Unfortunately, it is virtually impossible to design definitive research in a constantly shifting environment. When this study was first considered there were still relatively few hospices; by the time the study was being implemented, *hospice* was nearly a household word, and the number of organizations purportedly providing hospice care was nearly five hundred. The "moving target" of hospice care required a flexible approach to understanding the central policy questions, which made it difficult to meet the normal standards of statistical rigor.

Designing large, multiple-setting studies such as the NHS implies that there will be replication of the hospice model throughout the country. Unfortunately, there is no standard hospice model, and the state of our knowledge about what features of hospice care are most effective in achieving desired outcomes is inadequate. The causal line of reasoning is highly complex; numerous factors influence whether and how well patient goals are achieved. Good medical-care planning may be related to improved symptom control. On the other hand, symptom control may be dependent on well-trained volunteers who are available nearly around the clock to alert the health professionals when intervention is required. Fervor and excitement may radiate sufficiently such that patients feel in better control of their symptoms in the absence of specific measures. All of these explanations could be true to some extent; current knowledge and analytic experience make it virtually impossible to determine their individual contributions.

Were it possible to understand the various influences upon patient outcome and how they interact with one another, we still might not be able to adequately determine whether certain outcomes are superior in one group than in another. One of the principal deficits we face is measurement complexity. Patient function and symptom experience are relevant end points of treatment, and these constructs can be reliably measured. Less precise is the definition and measurement of quality of life. Presently, quality-of-life measurement is receiving considerable attention from a number of research groups. Numerous questions remain. Can we appreciate and measure subjective experiences contaminated by cultural factors and value judgments? Is there social consensus around those features of life experience that are most valued and therefore more desirable? How can we apply quality-of-life measures to other cultures that value aspects of life experience differently? If patients and families must tell us what is important to them, how does the researcher cope with the fact that many patients are no longer able or willing to respond to lengthy, intrusive interviews about their quality of life?

In a study such as the NHS, interpretation and communication of the results present additional challenges. The scientists charged with conducting such studies strive to formulate precise expressions of the research questions, which can be subjected to statistical analysis. The agenda of the scientist is to satisfy his or her scientific constituency as well as to answer the policy questions as completely as the data and study design allow. Policy analysts have a different constituency and are less interested in nuances and qualifications regarding the meaning of the study results. The cultural gap between the two groups, academic scientists and political policy makers, is wide. For policy makers, research is often the vehicle for justifying a politically desirable strategy. The scientists' goals include the desire to affect policy decisions but also recognition by the scientific community. If these goals converge, it is often an accident.

The issues facing hospices are those facing the larger health-care system. As such, the hospice movement provides an interesting case study of a rapidly evolving system that may be a bellwether for many of the challenges that will face the medical-care system in the United States and elsewhere over the next several decades.

References

Abert, J. G. 1979. Health evaluation. In *Program evaluation at HEW. Part I: Health*, ed. J. A. Abert, pp. 77–112. New York: Marcel Dekker.

Abt, C. 1975. The social costs of cancer. *Social Indicators Research* 2:175–90.

Adriaensen, H., Mattelaer, B., and Van de Walle, J. 1980. The treatment of cancer pain with analgesic drugs. *Belgian Congress of Anesthesiology* 31:203–9.

Andrews, G., Tennant, C., Hewson, D. M., and Valliant, G. E. 1978. Life event stress, social support, coping style and risk of psychological impairment. *Journal of Nervous Mental Diseases* 166:307–37.

Aronson, G. J. 1959. Treatment of the dying person. In *The meaning of death*, ed. H. Feifel, pp. 251–58. New York: McGraw-Hill.

Ball, J. 1976–77. Widow's grief: The impact of age and mode of death. *OMEGA: Journal of Death and Dying* 7:314–25.

Belsley, D. A., Kuh, E., and Welsch, R. E. 1980. *Regression diagnostics: Identifying influential data and sources of collinearity.* New York: John Wiley.

Benoliel, J. G., and Crowley, D. M. 1974. The patient in pain: New concepts. *American Cancer Society* 1–4.

Bloom, B., and Kissick, P. 1980. Home and hospital cost of terminal illness. *Medical Care* 18:560–64.

Bloom, J. R. 1982. Social support systems and cancer: A conceptual view. In *Psychosocial aspects of cancer,* ed. J. Cohen, J. W. Cullen, and L. R. Martin. New York: Raven Press.

Bloom, J. R., Ross, R. D., and Burnell, G. M. 1978. Effect of social support on patient adjustment following breast surgery. *Patient Counsel. Health Educ.* 1:50–59.

Bond, M. R. 1979a. Psychologic and emotional aspects of cancer pain. In *Advances in pain research and therapy,* ed. J. J. Bonica and V. Ventafridda, vol. 2, pp. 81–88. New York: Raven Press.

———. 1979b. Psychologic and psychiatric techniques for the relief of advanced cancer pain. In *Advances in pain research and therapy,* ed. J. J. Bonica and V. Ventafridda, vol. 2, pp. 215–22. New York: Raven Press.

Bonica, J. 1980. Introduction and cancer pain. In *Pain research publications: Association for research in nervous and mental disease,* ed. J. Bonica, vol. 2. New York: Raven Press.

Bornstein, P. E., Clayton, P. J., Halikas, J. A., Maurice, W. L., and Robins, E. 1973. The depression of widowhood after thirteen months. *British Journal of Psychiatry* 122:561–66.

Bowman, L. 1959. *The American funeral.* Washington, D.C.: Public Affairs Press.

Breznitz, S. 1983. *The denial of stress.* New York: International Universities Press.

Buckingham, R. W., and Lack, S. A. 1978. *First American hospice.* New Haven, Conn: Hospice, Inc.

Bunch, J. 1972. Recent bereavement in relation to suicide. *Journal of Psychosomatic Research* 16(5):361–66.

Calhoun, L. G., and Selby, J. W. 1985. Social responses to bereaved persons: An examination of social rules. *Research Record* 2:51–68.

Cancer Care Inc. 1973. *The impact of costs and consequences of catastrophic illness on patients and families.* New York: Cancer Care Inc.

Carey, R. G. 1979–80. Weathering widowhood: Problems and adjustments of the widowed during the first year. *OMEGA: Journal of Death and Dying* 10:163–74.

Cassel, E. J. 1976. The contribution of the social environment to host resistance. *American Journal of Epidemiology* 8(2):107–23.

————. 1982. The nature of suffering and the goals of medicine. *The New England Journal of Medicine* 306(11):639–45.

Cassileth, B. R. 1979. *The cancer patient: Social and medical aspects of care.* Philadelphia: Lea & Febiger.

Chapman, C. R. 1979. Psychologic and behavioral aspects of cancer pain. In *Advances in Pain Research and Therapy,* ed. J. J. Bonica and V. Ventafridda, vol. 2, pp. 45–56. New York: Raven Press.

Christensen, D. B. 1978. Drug-taking compliance: A review and synthesis. *Health Services Research* 13(2).

Clayton, P. J. 1982. Bereavement. In *Handbook of affective disorders,* ed. E. S. Paykel. London: Churchill Livingstone.

Clayton, P. J., and Darvish, H. S. 1979. Course of depressive symptoms following the stress of bereavement. In *Stress and Mental Disorder,* ed. J. E. Barrett, pp. 121–36. New York: Raven Press.

Clayton, P. J., Herjanic, M., Murphy, G. E., and Woodruff, L. 1974. Mourning and depression: Their similarities and differences. *Canadian Psychiatric Association Journal* 19:309–12.

Cohen, J. 1982. Response of the health care system to the psychosocial aspects of cancer. In *Psychosocial aspects of cancer,* ed. J. Cohen, J. W. Cullen, and L. R. Martin. New York: Raven Press.

Creek, L. 1982. A homecare hospice profile: Description, evaluation, and cost analysis. *Journal of Family Practice* 14:53–58.

Davis, M. S. 1971. Variation in patient's compliance with doctor's orders, medical practice and doctor-patient interaction. *Psychiatry and Medicine* 2(1):31–54.

Dohrenwend, B. S., and Dohrenwend, B. P. 1981. *Stressful life events and their contexts.* New York: Prodist.

Downs, A. 1966. *Inside bureaucracy.* Boston: Little, Brown, and Co.

Draper, N., and Smith, H. 1981. *Applied regression analysis.* 2nd ed. New York: John Wiley.

DuBois, P. M. 1980. *The hospice way of death.* New York: Human Sciences Press.

Elliot, G. R., and Eisdorfer, C., eds. 1982. *Stress and human health.* New York: Springer Publishing Co.

Engel, G. L. 1961. Is grief a disease? *Psychosomatic medicine* 11:18–22.

Erikson, E. H. 1982. *The life cycle completed.* New York: W. W. Norton & Co.

Farrell, J. J. 1982. The dying of death: Historical perspectives. *Death Education* 8:105–24.

Feifel, H. 1963. The taboo on death. *American Behavioral Scientist* 6:66–67.

Feifel, H., ed. 1959. *The meaning of death.* New York: McGraw-Hill.

Feldman, A. R., Kessler, L., Myers, M. H., and Naughton, M. D. 1986. The prevalence of cancer: Estimates based on the Connecticut tumor registry. *New England Journal of Medicine* 315(22):1394–97.

Follick, M. J., Zitter, R. I., and Kulich, R. J. n.d. Outpatient management of chronic pain. Unpublished.

Glick, I., Weiss, R., and Parkes, C. 1974. *The first year of bereavement.* New York: John Wiley & Sons.

Goldberg, R. J., and Mor, V. 1985. A survey of psychotropic use in terminal cancer patients. *Psychosomatics* 26(9):745–51.

Goldberg, R. J., Mor, V., Wiemann, M. C., Greer, D. S., and Hiris, J. 1986. Analgesic use in terminal cancer patients: Report from the National Hospice Study. *Journal of Chronic Diseases* 39(1):37–45.

Graham, S., Snell, L. M., Graham, J. B., and Ford, L. 1971. Social trauma in the epidemiology of cancer of the cervix. *Journal of Chronic Diseases* 24:711–15.

Gravely, B. 1980. *Financial and statistical evaluation of the hospice program at Church Hospital Corporation.* Richmond, Va.: Department of Health Administration, Medical College of Virginia.

Greene, P. E. 1984. The pivotal role of the nurse in hospice care. *Cancer* 34(4):204–5.

Greer, D. S., Mor, V., Sherwood, S., Morris, J. N., and Birnbaum, H. 1983. National Hospice Study analysis plan. *Journal of Chronic Diseases* 36(11):737–80.

Gusterson, F. R. 1977. Role of residential care in terminal illness. In *Pain: New perspectives in measurement and management,* ed. A. W. Harcus, R. Smith, and B. Whittle, pp. 134–37. London: Churchill Livingstone.

Haberman, S. J. 1982. Analysis of dispersion of multinomial responses. *Journal of the American Statistical Association* 77(379):568–80.

Haeuser, A. A., and Schwartz, F. S. 1980. Developing social work skills for work with volunteers. *Social Casework: The Journal of Contemporary Social Work* 595–601.

Hardy, T. K., and Pritchard, R. I. 1977. Physical distress suffered by terminal cancer patients in hospital. *Anaesthesia* 32:647–49.

Hayes-Bautista, D. E. 1976. Modifying the treatment: Patient control and medical care. *Soc. Sci. Med.* 10:233–38.

Henry, N. L. 1986. *Public administration and public affairs.* New York: Prentice-Hall.

Holland, J. 1973. Psychologic aspects of cancer. In *Cancer medicine,* ed. J. Holland and E. Frel, pp. 991–1021. Philadelphia: Lea & Febiger.

Holmes, T. H., and Rahe, R. H. 1967. The social readjustment rating scale. *Journal of Psychosomatic Research* 11:213–18.

Houston, B., and Holmes, D. 1974. Effect of avoidant thinking and reappraisal for coping with threat involving temporal uncertainty. *Journal of Personality and Social Psychology* 30:382–88.

Joint Commission on Accreditation of Hospitals (JCAH) 1984. The Hospice Project. Draft report of the W. K. Kellogg Foundation–funded project. Chicago.

Kane, R. L., Wales, J., Bernstein, L., Leibowitz, A., and Kaplan, S. 1984. A randomised controlled trial of hospice care. *The Lancet* 1:890–94.

Karnofsky, D. A., Abelman, W. H., Craver, L. F., and Burchenal, J. H. 1948. The use of nitrogen mustards in palliative treatments of carcinoma. *Cancer* 56:634–56.

Karnofsky, D. A., and Burchenal, J. D. 1949. The clinical evaluation of chemotherapeutic agents in cancer. In *Evaluation of chemotherapeutic agents,* ed. C. M. Macleod, pp. 191–205. Symposium held at New York Academy of Medicine, New York, 1948. Columbia University Press.

Kasper, A. M. 1959. The doctor and death. In *The meaning of death,* ed. H. Feifel, pp. 259–83. New York: McGraw-Hill.

Kassakian, M. G., Bailey, L. R., Rinker, M., Stewart, C. A., and Yates, J. W. 1979. The cost and quality of dying: A comparison of home and hospital. *Nurse Practitioner* 4:18–23.

Kastenbaum, R. 1975. Toward standards of care for the terminally ill. Part II. What standards exist today? *Omega: Journal of Death and Dying* 6:289–90.

———. 1986. *Death, society, and human experience.* 3rd ed. Columbus, Ohio: Merrill Publishing Co.

———. In press. *The psychology of death.* 2d ed. New York: Springer Publishing Co.

Katz, S., Ford, A. B., Moskowitz, R. W., Jackson, B. A., and Jaffe, M. W. 1963. Studies of illness in the aged: The index of ADL: A standardized measure of biological and psychosocial function. *Journal of the American Medical Association* 185: 914–19.

Kaufmann, W. 1959. Existentialism and death. In *The Meaning of death,* ed. H. Feifel, pp. 39–63. New York: McGraw-Hill.

Kay, L. L. 1981. A cost analysis of three hospice programs: Hillhaven Hospice, Kaiser-Permanente Hospice, Riverside Hospice. Los Angeles, Kaiser-Permanente Medical Care Program.

Kessler, R. 1979. Stress and social status, and psychological distress. *Journal of Health and Social Behavior* 20:259–73.

Kimberly, J. R., and Miles, R. H. 1980. *The organizational life cycle.* San Francisco: Jossey-Bass Publishers.

Kirscht, J. P. 1977. Communication between patients and physicians. *Annals of Internal Medicine* 86(4):499–501.

Kleinbaum, D. G., Kupper, L. L., and Morgenstern, H. 1982. *Epidemiologic research.* Belmont, Calif.: Lifetime Learning Publications.

Klerman, G. L., and Izen, J. E. 1977. The effects of bereavement and grief on physical health and general well-being. *Advances in Psychosomatic Medicine* 9:63–104.

Kohut, J. M., and Kohut, S. 1984. *Hospice: Caring for the terminally ill.* Springfield, Ill.: Charles C. Thomas Publisher.

Kübler-Ross, E. 1969. *On death and dying.* New York: Macmillan Publishing Co.

Lack, S., and Buckingham, R. 1978. *The first American hospice: Three years of home care.* New Haven, Conn.: Hospice, Inc.

Laliberte, L., and Mor, V. 1985. An examination of the relationship of reimbursement and organizational structure to the use of hospice volunteers. *The Hospice Journal* 1(1):21–44.

Lamers, W. M. 1986. Hospice care in North America. In *Cancer, stress, and death,* ed. S. B. Day, pp. 133–48. New York: Plenum.

Lilienfeld, A. M., Levin, M. L., and Kessler, I. I. 1972. *Cancer in the United States.* Cambridge, Mass.: Harvard University Press.

Lindemann, E. 1944. The symptomatology and management of acute grief. *American Journal of Psychiatry* 101:141–48.

Lipman, A. G. 1980. Drug therapy in cancer pain. *Cancer Nursing* 2:39.

———. 1982. Myths and misconceptions about narcotic analgesics. *Education and Training* 2:1–2.

Lunt, B., and Hillier, R. 1981. Terminal care: Present services and future priorities. *British Medical Journal* (Clinical Research) 283(6291):595–98.

Maddison, D. C., and Viola, A. 1968. The health of widows in the year following bereavement. *Journal of Psychosomatic Research* 12:297–306.

Maguire, P. 1976. The psychological and social sequelas of mastectomy. In *Modern perspectives in the psychiatric aspects of surgery,* ed. J. G. Howell, pp. 390–422. New York: Brunnker/Mazel.

Marris, P. 1958. *Widows and their families.* London: Routledge & Kegan Paul.

Martinson, I., Armstrong, G., Geis, D., et al. 1978. Home care for children dying of cancer. *Pediatrics* 62:106–13.

Maslach, C. 1976. Burned out. *Human Behavior* 5(9):16–22.

Melzack, R. 1974. Psychological concepts and methods of the control of pain. In *Advances in Neurology.* vol. 4. New York: Raven Press.

Mitchell, G. W., and Glicksman, H. S. 1977. Cancer patients: Knowledge and attitudes. *Cancer* 40:61–66.

Mitford, J. 1963. *The American way of death.* New York: Simon and Schuster.

Mor, V. 1984. Data collection methodology and instruments of the National Hospice Study. NTIS PB-84-188911.

Mor, V., and Hiris, J. 1983. Determinants of site of death among hospice cancer patients. *Journal of Health and Social Behavior* 24:375–85.

Mor, V., and Laliberte, L. 1984. Burnout among hospice staff. *Health and Social Work* 9(4):274–83.

Mor, V., Laliberte, L., Morris, J. N., and Wiemann, M. C. 1984. The Karnofsky Performance Status Scale: An examination of its reliability and validity in a research setting. *Cancer* 53(9):2002–7.

Mor, V., Schwartz, R., Laliberte, L., and Hiris, J. 1985. An examination of the effect of reimbursement and organizational structure on the allocation of hospice staff time. *Home Health Care Services Quarterly* 6(1):101–18.

Mor, V., Wachtel, T. J., and Kidder, D. 1985. Patient predictors of hospice choice: Hospital versus home care programs. *Medical Care* 23(9):1115–19.

Morris, J. N., Mor, V., Goldberg, R. J., Sherwood, S., Greer, D. S., and Hiris, J. 1986. The effect of treatment setting and patient characteristics on pain in terminal cancer patients: A report from the National Hospice Study. *Journal of Chronic Diseases* 39(1):27–35.

Morris, J. N., Suissa, S., Wright, S., Sherwood, S., and Greer, D. 1986. Last days: A study of the quality of life of terminally ill cancer patients. *Journal of Chronic Diseases* 39(1):47–62.

Mount, B. M. 1976. The problem of caring for the dying in a general hospital: The palliative care unit as a possible solution. *Canadian Medical Association Journal* 115(2):119–21.

Murphy, G. 1959. Discussion. In *The meaning of death*, ed. H. Feifel, pp. 317–40. New York: McGraw-Hill.

National Center for Health Statistics 1982. Advance report of final mortality statistics, 1979. *Monthly Vital Statistics Report* 31(6).

National Hospice Organization 1981. *Standards of a hospice program of care*. McClean, Va.: National Hospice Organization.

National Hospice Organization 1985. *Hospice News* 3(1).

New York State Department of Health 1982. An analysis and evaluation of the New York State hospice demonstration program. Albany.

Paradis, L. F. 1983. The integration of hospice programs into the traditional health care system. Doctoral dissertation: Michigan State University.

Paradis, L. F. 1984. Hospice program integration: An issue for policymakers. *Death Education* 8(5–6):383–98.

Parkes, C. M. 1965. Bereavement and mental illness, part 1: A clinical study of the grief of bereaved psychiatric patients. *British Journal of Medical Psychology* 38:1–12.

Parkes, C. M., and Brown, R. 1972. Health and bereavement: A controlled study of Boston widows and widowers. *Psychosomatic Medicine* 34:449–61.

Patchner, M. A., and Finn, M. B. 1987–88. Volunteers: The life-line of hospice. *Omega: Journal of Death and Dying* 18(2).

Rando, T. A. 1986. A comprehensive analysis of anticipatory grief: Perspectives, processes, promises, and problems. In *Loss and anticipatory grief*, ed. T. A. Rando, pp. 3–38. Lexington, Mass.: D. C. Heath and Co.

Raphael, B. 1983. *The anatomy of bereavement*. New York: Basic Books.

Reuben, D. B., and Mor, V. 1986. Dyspnea in terminal cancer patients. *Chest* 89(2):234–36.

Rice, D. P. 1966. *Estimating the cost of illness*. Health Economics Series No. 6, PHS Pub. No. 947–6, Washington, D.C.: U.S. Government Printing Office.

Rosenblatt, P. C. 1983. *Bitter, bitter tears*. Minneapolis: University of Minnesota Press.

Sanders, C. M. 1977. Typologies and symptoms of adult bereavement. Doctoral dissertation, Tampa: University of South Florida.

Saunders, C. 1967. *The management of terminal illness*. London: Hospital and Medicine Publications Ltd.

———. 1976. Control of pain in terminal cancer. *Nursing Times* 72:1133–35.

———. 1978. Hospice care. *American Journal of Medicine* 65(5):726–28.

———. 1981. The hospice: Its meaning to patients and their physicians. *Hospital Practice* 93–108.

Shimm, D. S., Logue, D. L., Maltbie, A. A., and Dugan, S. 1979. Medical management of chronic cancer pain. *Journal of the American Medical Association* 241:2408–12.

Siegler, I. C., and Costa, P. T. 1985. Health behavior relationships. In *Handbook of the psychology of aging*, ed. J. E. Birren and K. W. Schaie, pp. 144–68. New York: Van Nostrand Reinhold.

Spitzer, W. O., Dobson, A. J., Hall, J., Chesterman, E., Levi, J., Shepherd, R., Battista, R., and Catchlove, B. R. 1981. Measuring the quality of life of cancer patients: A concise QL index for use by physicians. *Journal of Chronic Diseases* 34:585–97.

Stannard, D. E. 1977. *The Puritan way of death*. New York: Oxford University Press.

Stedeford, A. 1979. Psychotherapy of the dying patient. *British Journal of Psychiatry* 135:7–14.

Stoddard, S. 1978. *Hospice movement—A better way of caring for the dying*. New York: Stein and Day.

Switzer, D. K. 1970. *The dynamics of grief*. Nashville, Tenn.: Abingdon Press.

Symonds, P. 1977. Methadone in the elderly (letter). *British Medical Journal* 1(6059):512.

Taylor, J. 1651. *The rules and exercises of holy dying*. Reprinted 1977. New York: Arno Press.

Theorell, T. 1974. Life events before and after the onset of a premature myocardial infarction. In *Stressful life events: Their nature and effects*, ed. B. S. Dohrenwood and B. P. Dohrenwood, pp. 101–17. New York: John Wiley & Sons.

Turk, D. C., and Rennert, K. 1981. Pain and the terminally ill cancer patient: A cognitive-social learning perspective. In *Behavior therapy in terminal care: A humanistic approach*, ed. H. J. Sobel. Cushing Hospital Series on Aging and Terminal Care, eds. R. J. Kastenbaum and T. X. Barber. Cambridge, Mass.: Ballinger Publishing Company.

Twycross, R. G. 1977. Choice of strong analgesic in terminal cancer: Diamorphine or morphine? *Pain* 3(2):93–104.

———. 1979. The Brompton Cocktail. In *Advances in pain research and therapy*, eds. J. J. Bonica and V. Ventafridda. Vol. 2. New York: Raven Press.

———. 1984. *Pain relief and cancer*. Philadelphia: Saunders Publishing Company.

Twycross, R. G., and Lack, S. A. 1984. *Therapeutics in terminal cancer*. London: Pitman Publishing, Ltd.

Vachon, M. L. S. 1976. Grief and bereavement following the death of a spouse. *Canadian Psychiatric Association Journal* 21:35–44.

Vachon, M. L. S., Sheldon, A. R., Lancee, W. J., Lyall, W. A. L., Rogers, J., and Freeman, S. J. J. 1982. Correlates of enduring distress patterns following bereavement: Social network, life situation and personality. *Psychosomatic Medicine* 12:783–88.

Veatch, R. M., and Tai, E. 1980. Talking about death: Patterns of lay and professional change. *Ann. Am. Acad. Pol. Soc. Sci.* 447:29–45.

Wachtel, T. J., and Mor, V. 1985. The use of transfusion in terminal cancer patients: Hospice versus conventional care setting. *Transfusion* 25(3):278–79.

Walsh, T. D., and Saunders, C. M. 1981. Oral morphine for relief of chronic pain from cancer. *New England Journal of Medicine* 305:1417–18.

Waugh, E. 1948. *The loved one*. Boston: Little, Brown, & Co.

Weber, M. 1947. *The theory of social and economic organizations.* New York: Scribner's.

Weiner, A., Gerber, I., Battin, D., and Arkin, A. M. 1975. The process and phenomenology of bereavement. In *Bereavement: Its psychosocial aspects,* eds. B. Schoenberg, I. Berger, A. Weiner, and A. H. Kutcher. New York: Columbia University Press.

Weisman, A. D. 1972. *On death and denying.* New York: Behavioral Publications, Inc.

Weisman, A., Worden, J., and Sobel, H. 1980. Psychosocial screening and intervention with cancer patients. Research report of Project Omega, Boston, Massachusetts.

Wolf, M. H., Putnam, S. M., James, S. A., and Stiles, W. B. 1978. The medical interview satisfaction scale: Development of a scale to measure patient perceptions of physician behavior. *Journal of Behavioral Medicine* 1:391–401.

Yalom, I. 1977. Group therapy with the terminally ill. *American Journal of Psychiatry* 134:396–400.

Zimmerman, J. 1981. *Hospice: Complete care for the terminally ill.* Baltimore: Urban and Schwarzenberg.

Index

261

alternatives in, x, 2, 9, 187
costs of, 2, 55–62
and interpersonal relationships, 9, 10
and Medicare, 12
and naturalism, 14
and pain reduction, 9, 10
role of federal government in, ix, 2, 12
traditional, x, 2, 10
Therapists, 21, 71
Time, 5, 7
Treatment
See also Pain, control of
aggressive therapies, 89, 90–93, 234, 246
diagnostic testing, 89, 93–95, 238
intravenous intervention, 102, 108, 238
medication in, 99–102, 108, 120
respiratory therapy, 96–98
and social services, 89
supportive-palliative services in, xii, 12,
89, 95–99, 133, 228, 234, 237, 238,
243
"Treatment of the Dying Person" (Aronson),
5

Veterans Administration hospitals, 104
Viola, A., 152
Visiting Nurse Association, 17, 18

Volunteers, 187–208, 210, 244, 246
See also *specific types of hospices*
activities of, 20, 33, 45, 193–96
commitment of, 209, 249
description of hospice, 189–93
future of, 205–6, 227, 228, 238, 239
and home care, 17–18
in hospital hospices, 17
in independent hospices, 18
liability insurance for, 206
motives of, 191
number of hours spent by, 197–200, 207
nurse, 190–91, 196
vs. professional staff, ix–xi, 21, 201
and public policy, 231, 250
ratio of, to paid staff, 201–5, 207, 213,
222, 224, 225
social-service, 104

Waugh, Evelyn, *Loved One,* 6
Weber, M., 210
Weisman, Avery D., 151
Weiss, R., 152

Zimmerman, J., 194–95